Long Days, Last Days . . .
a down-to-earth guide
for those at the bedside

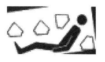

Hillel Schwartz

Long Days, Last Days . . .

a down-to-earth guide for those at the bedside

Cover image: Study of Hands, by Leonardo da Vinci
Codex Windsor, from a photograph in the public domain
http://commons.wikimedia.org/wiki/
File:Leonardo_da_Vinci_-_Study_of_hands_-_WGA12812.jpg

ISBN-13 978-1482785777
ISBN-10 1482785773

In memory of
Anne, Ben, Connie, Donald,
Esther, Ferdinand, Fritzie,
Hank, Harry, Minnie, Steve

and for Sid and Suzanne

TABLE of CONTENTS

TABLE OF CONTENTS, continued

TABLE OF CONTENTS, continued

TABLE OF CONTENTS, continued

TABLE OF CONTENTS, continued

At Any Given Moment: A Forward

At any given moment, five million people on this planet are at the bedsides of grandparents, parents, wives, husbands, lovers, friends, or children who are seriously, perhaps incurably, ill. Some 200,000 are at the bedsides of those who are dying-- in pain or oblivious, anxious or at peace. This book is not for the Departing; it is for the many who will be staying on but who must be, who want to be, at the bedside.

And not just once. Most of us will be at the bedside time and again. In the last twelve years I have been called to seven bedsides as a son, a lover, a close friend. As a case manager, I have been called to many other bedsides.

Before the advent of antibiotics, transfusions, and dialysis, the Last Days were usually brief; often now they are extended, sometimes comfortably, sometimes grotesquely. At no time, however, was it common for the Last Days to resemble those scenes in paintings, novels, or films where families gather around a dying person to receive moral instruction and make fond farewells. Worldwide, more people still die at home or in war zones (or post-disaster tent-camps) than in medical settings, but nowhere can one count on the Last Days being well-spoken or heartwarming.

In the United States, three-quarters of the Departing die of complications arising from chronic conditions: heart, lung, or kidney disease; diabetes; recurrent cancer; AIDS; dementia. Such conditions, with their associated regimes of capsules, injections, infusions, or radiation, often narrow a person's capacity to ponder, perceive, respond, share. With new drugs, advanced surgical techniques, and more effective protocols of intensive care, once-fatal strokes and heart attacks are now preludes, later or sooner, to chronic debility and a gradual loss of competence.

The upshot is that it is harder to tell when Long Days may be turning toward Last Days. So all of us will be spending more time at complicated bedsides in hospitals, rehabilitation units, skilled nursing facilities, assisted living complexes, board-and-care establishments, or back home. As the rhythms of physical and mental decline have become less steady, so the tempos of dying have become more indeterminate, and unsettling.

Would that we could be better prepared. We struggle at each bedside for the clarity, knowledge, energy, and emotional strength to cope with the Long and Last Days of a loved one, and it seems no easier on the third or fourth go-around. At any given moment, what do we say? When is it best to keep still? to talk quietly? to speak up? At difficult moments, what do we do? When is it best to do nothing? to quietly make things happen? to act forcefully, directly?

Spiritual traditions have parables and songs on how to die well, prayers and rituals for mourning. Hospital social workers have in-house guides, as do funeral directors. There are manuals for palliative care and end-of-life nursing. Hospices publish brochures for clients and syllabi for volunteers. So abundant are the published accounts of the last years and days of loved ones that a librarian could sort such books by disease, by location (hospital, assisted living, home), or by the nature of the relationship (twins? old friends? former lovers? mentor and student?).

Few are the pages devoted to those at the bedside and what they can expect during Long Days and Last Days. This book is for them.

That is, for *us*, in our millions. For those of us coping month after month with loved ones who have serious or terminal illnesses but are not yet in their Last Days. For those of us at the bedside who feel harassed, angry, exhausted, or at sea on the approach of the Last Days. Finally, for those of us who have been through a recent departure and have begun reflecting on what we went through.

This book is also for the nurses, caregivers, and counselors who seek to appreciate the perspective and experiences of those at the bedside as Long Days become Last Days. And for the therapists, physicians, social workers, and hospice staff who are regularly asked for advice on how to deal with the messy issues that arise.

Each chapter addresses one of those issues. You will see by the headings that some chapters are blunt, others double-edged, metaphorical. Several topics you may already have broached; others will come as a surprise. In any case, each chapter is intended to give you a handle on a certain situation, a context by which to make sense of a series of events, prospects from which to confront a quandary, frames through which to address a sharp or subtle uneasiness.

At Any Given Moment, continued

Most chapters can be read in five minutes or less. The chapters are arranged alphabetically so that you can find topics swiftly and handily. Some readers will choose to go through the chapters *p.r.n., pro re nata*, "as circumstances arise." Others may work through the alphabet prospectively, in anticipation of circumstances not yet arisen. At the back I provide short lists for Further Reading and Viewing and a set of useful websites.

Caution: This is not a book for those who must be at the bedside of dying infants and young children. Others, better informed, write about this.

Myself, I come to Long Days and Last Days from six directions. First, as a scholar of millenarian movements, where the Last Days are imagined in charged terms as both catastrophe and revelation, and for which dramatic scenarios are ever rewritten. Next, as an historian of medicine who has studied changes in attitudes toward the dying, improbable advances in technology, shifts in methods of diagnosis and philosophies of prognosis, rethinkings of the definition and management of pain. Next, as the lover of a woman who spent ten years coping with chemotherapy, radiation treatments, mastectomies, and horrendous pain from breast cancer that metastasized to the bones and killed her. Next, as the son of a father who fought a harrowing battle against prostate cancer and died in the eleventh year of that campaign. Next, as case manager for an old friend who had to deal with two strokes caused by an underlying cancer, and who needed more help than could be provided even by three accomplished adult children. All this led me to co-found, with Melissa McCool, a psychiatric social worker, Sage Case Management, whose philosophy may be reviewed at www.sagecase.com.

So this handbook is drawn from direct and deep experience with one person after another, one family after another, year after year, for twenty years. I make no false promises about ease. Instead, I offer tools that you may find useful *at the bedside*: questions to ask of physicians, of the Departing, of yourself; technical details you may need to grasp; emotional, familial, and philosophical preparations you may need to make. *Long Days, Last Days* has nothing to do with deathbed conversions on either side of the handrails; it has much to do with conversations along the way, and with accomplished gifts of silence, of thoughtfulness and tenderness.

7 WAYS TO USE THIS BOOK

1. Foregrounding (A-Z). During the Long Days or in anticipation of the Last Days, whether as a caregiver, a counselor, a good friend, a spouse, parent, or child, you read this book through, unhurriedly, from beginning to end, for perspective on what will be asked of you and others. Some parts you read aloud to those who will be partners at the bedside, and some perhaps to the Departing.

2. For Grounding (e.g., Checklists, Keepsakes, Lawyers, Pain, Respite): During the Long Days or on the approach of the Last Days, you read to gain your footing, searching out those sections that you suspect will prove personally most useful.

3. Foresight: (Advocacy: Gatekeeping: Moths and Ministering Angels): You pick out a chapter of immediate interest and follow the internal hyperlinks so as to appreciate the ramifications.

4. For Insight (Details, Holding on, Mothers and Fathers): Puzzled or disturbed by some events or recurrent thoughts, you look for specific chapters that help put these in context.

5. Foregoing (Strength but not Cascades; Last Things but not Last Breaths): Amid the turmoil and fatigue of the Long and Last Days, you turn to pages for relief or confirmation; other chapters just now are too disconcerting, so you pass them by.

6. For the Going Off (Funeral Arrangements, Last Words, Veterans): Just before a departure, you select chapters that deal with what will happen now, what needs to be arranged, what may happen next.

7. Retrospection (Z-A): Weeks or months later, you begin to reflect on your days at the bedside, wanting to make sense of what transpired, for in the near future there will be other calls to the bedside, other departures. Then you happen upon this book, which perhaps someone gave you during the Last Days but which you had not opened, could not bear the thought of. Now it looks interesting, and you start at the end, as would be fitting, with Zero Visibility.

For additional resources, see Further Reading, Further Viewing, and Useful Websites

Note: An arrow → indicates that the next word has its own dedicated chapter. {Brackets} reference related chapters.

ABSOLUTES

No absolutes.

Nothing in this book is meant to be taken as an imperative or an unswerving truth.

No absolutes: in spiritual traditions, death itself is no absolute. Across the continents, rites of remembrance or rituals of release argue that death is less than final, more than another farewell.

Still, no one anywhere welcomes a long debilitating decline, and few welcome a lingering or painful or stutter-step death.

And we may →grieve as much before a death as afterward.

For those of us who live within hand's grasp of another's Long or Last Days, within arm's reach we find nurses, physicians, counselors, therapists, and men and women of the cloth, not to mention lawyers, accountants, seers, soothsayers, and life coaches. They each share what wisdom, skill, and empathy they have.

This book concerns what all of them tend to overlook-- because too awkward or picayune, too obnoxious or obvious, too unmanageable or indeterminate.

Those things, in other words, that together make up each messy moment of our own ongoing lives, and the lives of the Departing, during Long Days and Last Days.

ACCIDENTALS

A term from philosophy: that which is merely incidental to one's being. There are accidents, and there are essences. A person may have long nails or short nails--those are accidents of diet, of culture, of fashion, of occupation. But what is a human being without a heart, lungs, brain?

You think that a person in the Last Days is remorselessly shaking off or shedding accidentals, the way one throws off one's clothes as one runs into the ocean, stripping down to bare essentials. Each day you find the Departing less interested in the weather, less invested in the news, or less stirred by a favorite song. It is much harder to please him with what once pleased him. It is harder to prove to her, by showing that you know what pleases her, that you love her regardless of what she looks like now, thinner or weaker, unfocused or half-asleep. And isn't this a sign that the Long Days are turning toward the Last Days?

The body too suddenly has accidentals, parts that until recently could only have been essences, now being sloughed off or slipping away. How can anyone do without so much? Who is this person now, and how shall I recognize her, how shall I embrace him? {→Identity.} Do the dying dream, or are dreams too just accidentals?

In the company of such a severe stripping down, you tend to blame yourself for being still preoccupied with things that loom large in your mind today but have nothing to do with life and death, with essences. How foolish to worry about car payments or the price of gas or a ragged fingernail. What does it really matter if there is famine in India (isn't there always famine in India?) or childhood poverty in Detroit and Rio de Janeiro (isn't there always?) . . . . Don't you owe it to this person in the Last Days to do your damnedest to focus on the basics?

Funny thing: a person does not give up on accidentals just because these are the Last Days. Dearest accidentals may themselves be incidental to the bedclothes or the room or the season, but until the end, or until opiates cloud the end, things often stick.

So it is not *only human* but truly human, while you are keeping company during the Long Days and →Last Days, to have thoughts less than noble, memories ignoble, and to stand each morning before your wardrobe considering lines and colors.

The dying do not expect us to die alongside them.

ACUTENESS

How do you know that a situation is medically "acute"?
How do you know when to call 911? {→Urgency}?
Will you lose standing for "crying wolf"?

Unless a →Do Not Resuscitate (DNR) order is in effect,
act immediately when a person
1) cannot breathe
2) is choking, or looks to be swallowing the tongue
3) is swelling up quickly and in danger of choking
4) has suddenly lost the capacity to smile or speak coherently
5) suddenly cannot move a leg or raise an arm
6) is doubled over in pain that does not relent in a few minutes
7) is screaming in →delirium and likely to hurt others or self
8) has blacked out and appears unconscious
9) has extreme vertigo and is on the floor
10) has unremitting nausea and →vomiting
11) is bleeding profusely (except perhaps from the nose)
12) has a bone or organ protruding from the skin.

Facing any of the above, your first inclination would surely be
to call 911 and then to apply what you know of first aid (the
Heimlich maneuver, an Epipen, rescue inhalers, a tourniquet).
Even with a DNR, all warrant an urgent call to a physician,
because DNRs never preclude keeping a person comfortable.
For example, bones can be set without violating a DNR.

And rest assured, no one would upbraid you for "crying wolf" on
any of these. (Also rest assured, most communities and
insurance plans pay for ambulances in an emergency.)

However, if at home at the bedside during Long Days and Last
Months, there will be much that you will be expected to do with
drugs or devices on hand: →oxygen (for 1, 8), tongue
depressors (2), pain pills, drops, or pumps (6, 7), Antivert or
Meclizine (9), Xanax or Zofran (10). Acuteness then takes on a
different cast, for at issue is rather the acuteness of your
judgment than the acuteness of an episode which is one in a
series to which most at the bedside have grown accustomed.

As you come to manage "acute" situations on your own, one
danger is that you will medically and emotionally downgrade
the "acute" to "routine" while the bedridden person lives in
ever-greater dread of yet another recurrence of breakthrough
pain or explosive vomiting. Your newfound confidence should
not obscure the fact of excruciating attacks upon the body and
psyche of the person you came to sit beside. However much
the acute has died down to routine for you, it is never less than
acute for him, or her.

ADVOCACY

One of those lines that is hardest to draw: how much to speak on behalf of the Departing, how much to solicit their opinions, how much to accept their silences. The West is so committed to definitions of personhood centered upon will, willfulness, willpower, and won't-power (the power to say NO), that we look toward →Wills and prior →Directives not only to protect but to constitute a person in extremity {→Identity}.

Last wishes seem so definitive of a person that they become sacrosanct, in part because they have usually been deliberated and declared well before, as if it is not the dying that is writ in stone but the will that anticipates the dying. How much can we allow the Departing to change their minds during the Last Days? How much do we attribute any changes of mind to the circumstances of dying, and for that reason downplay or dismiss them: "it's the drugs talking"; "she's out of her mind with pain"; "he can't remember much of anything."

So advocacy, which would seem to be one of the inarguable obligations of those at the bedside, demands a continual reconsideration of purpose and prospect. Of purpose: am I advocating on behalf of the person before me this instant, or of the person a week ago, a year ago? Of prospect: am I advocating for the moment (what the Departing requires now), or in the attributive conditional (this is what he would want) or in retrospect (this is what she would have wanted)?

And for whom am I an advocate? For myself (I cannot bear seeing her treated this way; I cannot stand the →noise in this hospital)? For others coming in from out of town (J. will be devastated if she gets here too late; K. will be upset with the mess that the doctors have made). For the Departing as he was a year or two ago? as she was before the decline?

Whatever else advocacy is, in some inevitable measure it is an act of projection backward or forward in time, there or anywhere-but-here. It is also a projection of myself--my exhaustion, my heightened sensitivities, my desire for solace-- onto the Departing, which we might call empathy.

Yet the Departing do need advocates, sometimes for the simplest of things (chips of ice, a drawn blind, new bed linen), sometimes against the most difficult of people (a meddling hospice nurse, an officious chaplain, all others who presume to speak omnisciently for the seriously ill and the Departing).

The longer you are at the bedside during the Long and Last Days, the more likely that advocacy becomes unavoidable. Can it also be clear-headed, resolute, wise?

AGEING

How old is old? Who is "getting on in years," who is "elderly"?

Sixty-five no longer entails retirement; "senior" no longer entails a move to a "retirement home." Ageing is conditioned as much by historical and psychosocial circumstance as by physiology, and the experience of ageing differs by gender, genetics, income, and degree of isolation or engagement.

"Senility" in its original sense simply meant growing old. That we now take it to refer to a loss of mental and physical capacity reflects rather a modern emphasis on youth and athleticism than some inevitable biology of ageing. Not everyone who grows old becomes senile, although a decline of short-term memory may well accompany advances into very old age--my uncle began noticing this when he rounded the corner on 102.

Then there is the opposite, premature senility. We joke about "senior moments," but premature senility is a terrifying oxymoron not gentled by diagnosis of "early onset Alzheimer's."

Our media now conflate ageing, dementia, →forgetfulness, and feebleness with a syndrome identified by Alois Alzheimer in 1906. Since we have as yet no effective treatments to stop, let alone reverse, the progression of Alzheimer's, its darker aspects loom over ageing even as we have shunted old age from the 60s into the 80s. This, notwithstanding a club for centenarians in Florida that requires new members to stand on their heads.

What are the repercussions for the bedside? Well, we are more easily shocked when younger people contract illnesses or incur injuries we associate with the aged. Vice versa, once a happily active, mentally alert "senior" becomes seriously ill, we tend to interpret his cognitive glitches and her physical complaints as much in terms of an underlying, untreatable senility as in terms of the diagnosed, treatable illness. Finally, the older a patient, the less we expect a full recovery; this lowering of expectation shows in our faces if not in the panorama of our services.

Philosophically, ageing returns us to question of →accidents and essences. How much of who I am is defined by what I can do physically and sexually, by how well I can remember or reason? Even were I to accept the postulate that my essence is immaterial, how do I express that ongoing essence otherwise than through my physical self, my words, my touch? Does debilitating illness or the onset of Departure so change things that I become either inaccessible or a kind of impostor? And who do you think you are, at my bedside? You too are ageing, and changing, and becoming someone you never were.

AGENCIES

Contracting with an agency to provide paid caregivers at home is rarely a first step during Long Days or Last Months. Before making this decision, you have likely tried out more informal, familial, or collegial arrangements. Once you find these too chancy or exhausting (→Mutual Peril) and particularly once it's clear that long-term care will be needed, then all concerned must still scrutinize the finances to determine whether paid care is feasible.

Since neither Medicare nor private health insurance other than long-term care policies will cover the expenses of non-medical help, and since the hourly rate of caregivers ranges from $15-$25, with a live-in daily rate of $150-$300+, the decision to work with an agency is consequential, as annual bills for full-time care can run to $75,000. This is more, sometimes much more, than the cost of a reasonable Assisted Living or board-and-care establishment ($3500-$6000+ a month). Note: bills now up before Congress would establish a minimum wage for live-in caregivers that could significantly increase the daily rate.

If you decide on home care, here are Questions to Ask of Agencies:

Agency background:
• How long have you been in business?
• Do you belong to any regional or state associations?
• Are any of the owners or managers MDs? RNs?
• Do you have a medical (home health) arm?
• Do you have someone on-call 24-7?
• Do you assure immediate substitutes in case of caregiver
    illness or other emergency?
• Other:_ _

Financial issues {and see also →Caregivers--Hiring}
• What are the daily live-in rates?
• Are holiday rates higher? If so, which holidays?
• Do you charge for care during days when the client is in
    a hospital, SNF, or rehab unit?
• Do hours worked begin when a caregiver enters the home?
• Is there a contract, a service agreement, or...?
• How, and how quickly, can services be terminated?
    Is there a fee for terminating?
• Do you require a deposit?
• How often do you bill? Can you bill electronically?
• Other:_ _

AGENCIES, continued

Caregiver background:
• How many caregivers do you employ?
• Are they bonded?
• How do you screen them?
  • National check for criminal records, bankruptcy, warrants?
  • Drug screening?
  • References?
• Are any of your caregivers otherwise licensed as CNAs, etc.?
• Do you give your caregivers special training in first aid?
• Are your caregivers fluent speakers of English?
• Do you have any caregivers fluent in [language of interest]?
• Can we interview caregivers in person? at the home?
    {and see→Caregivers--Interviewing}
• Other:_ _

Caregiver duties and services:
• What services are your caregivers prepared to perform?
        •Bathing/Showering? •Toileting? •Cleaning? •Cooking?
        •Laundry? •Errands? •Emptying catheter or ostomy bags?
        •Wrapping bandages and replacing dressings?
• What services are your caregivers not allowed to perform?
        •Organizing/administering meds? •Helping with nebulizers?
        •Injections? •Helping with home dialysis? •Wound care?
• Do your caregivers maintain a daily memorandum sheet?
• Do they bring their own meals?
• Do they all have working cell phones?
    • Once hired, are we allowed to call them directly?
• Are caregivers insured to use their own cars to drive clients to
    • medical appointments?
    • shopping and browsing?
    • movies, plays, excursions?
    • If so, is there a mileage charge?
• How many hours of uninterrupted sleep do live-ins require?
• Must they have their own bedroom? Own bathroom?
• How many days off must they have each week?
    • How do you arrange shifts among caregivers?
    • Who determines the time that each shift begins?
• Other:_ _

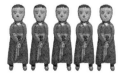

AIRLINES

Airlines offer Bereavement or Compassionate Fares for those who must travel at the last minute to the bedside of a family member who is gravely ill. {→Overnight Bags.} These fares can be booked within hours of a flight and allow for stays of up to a month, sometimes with no fee for changing the return date. Most airlines issue these fares over the phone; a few require the purchase to be made in person at the airport.

You will need to provide:
1. Name of the person who is ill or dying.
2. Your relationship to that person (acceptable: grandparent, parent, spouse, child, grandchild, aunt, uncle, brother, sister, niece, nephew, step-parent or sister and, usually, legal guardian, same-sex domestic partner, clergy).
3. Name, address and phone number of the hospital or other facility, as appropriate, and the name of an institutional contact.
4. Name and contact number of the attending physician (and, for a few airlines, a copy of hospital admission/discharge papers or a doctor's letter).
If you are flying to a funeral, 3 and 4 are different:
3. Name, address and phone number of the mortuary/funeral home, and contact person there.
4. Date of the burial and/or memorial service.

If you are too distressed to do this up front, you may instead apply for a refund, based upon what the Bereavement Fare would have been for the flights you did take, within ninety days after completing your trip. You will need to show receipts, boarding passes and, if you have returned from a funeral, a death certificate or letter from the mortuary.

Bereavement fares for international travel are less easily obtained and ordinarily are granted only as refunds upon your return, with proof of death in hand.

If you are already en route elsewhere and must change flights to get to the bedside, airlines may assist with free standby.

Amtrak and some bus services also have Bereavement Fares. El Al has a special department that helps with arrangements for transport for burial in Israel. For more details, check:
www.ehow.com/how_5879468_bereavement air fare.html
www.hotwire.com/bereavement.jsp
http://airtravel.about.com/lr/bereavement_airfares/441519/2/
www.funeralnet.com/info_guide/tra_index.html

ANNIVERSARIES

This comes up more often than you might think.

During Long Days and Last Days, and in more than one conversation, you compare ages at which people had their first heart attacks or how many years they lived with cancer or kidney failure. {→Dialysis.} You re-count to yourself and perhaps to others the age at death of a sister or husband and the age of the Departing. You make a roster of the dead, the dying, and those still going strong. Then, naturally, you cross-check your own age against that roster. Are you younger or older than the age at which your father passed away, your mother had a stroke, your older brother was hit by a car and almost died, your older sister had her chemotherapy? →Sitting at the bedside, you have time to go back several generations with this cross-check, and sometimes you do, looking for patterns, or milestones, or fate.

The seriously ill and the Departing do this too.

Approaching anniversaries can be scary. That sentence is properly ambiguous. And improperly ambiguous: for is it proper to be considering the scale of your own life when you are in the presence of, and hoping to be actively present to, someone in the Last Days? How dare you spend this precious time listing, under your breath, your own narrow escapes, or fantasizing about the breath of relief you are going to draw when you make it past the ages at which your parents or siblings died?

The older the Departing is, the longer your roster and the greater the chance of finding a pattern that goes to the heart of some matter that is more likely yours at the bedside than hers in the bed. But the older the Departing is, the greater the local solace and public celebration of the age he has reached ("a full life," "a natural end") and, conversely, the more terrifying for you the number of anniversary deaths you must make it past to arrive at anywhere near her age. {→Ageing}

That we are all mortal is, in this context, no consolation. That we know we are mortal, yet go on risking ourselves for others, and accompanying them at the end, may be.

ANSWERING MACHINES

These are almost obsolete, so I treat them as figures of speech.

What message should be put on an answering machine during Long and Last Days?
__Thanks for calling, but please don't leave a message; call Z.
__I am in the hospital/hospice/etc.
__[Default prerecorded message that came with the machine.]

As figures of speech, Answering Machines pose questions:
1. How engaged does a person want to be in Long/Last Days?
2. What kind of responsiveness do you expect of that person?
3. What counts as a response?

These are all troubling questions. After all, aren't you at the bedside because you know that your own immediate presence matters to her, his presentness to you?

We have powerful expectations--religious, literary, ethical--that those cognizant of an approaching end should spend their time and remaining energies on people and things that matter most. Wouldn't it violate some rule of decorum were the Departing to watch soap operas all day instead of talking with →brothers and sisters, children, you? Aren't you deferring the business of your own life in order to honor her during this ultimate transition? How can the Last Days be meaningful if the Departing insists on taking the calls of telephone marketers?

Or what if the seriously ill, whether or not on the verge of the Last Days, takes no calls, entertains no conversations, not even yours. What are you going to do if these Long Days are days of blankness, silence, restless sleep, or obsessive wrestling with sudoku puzzles? What are you yourself looking for by way of a persuasive communion? What is the person in the bed looking for?

Very close to the end, the →eyes turn away or upward or off into space, sometimes wandering, sometimes staring or searching. Up to that point, close calm quiet company may be all that is wanted. After that, to insist upon your own presence, to demand a response, is →selfish, obtrusive. And yet . . . .

The tactile and the auditory are ordinarily the last of the senses to go {→Hearing / Voices}. Even in great pain, in twilight sleep, words may be heard, a touch may be felt. Imminent departure is not death; absence of response is not necessarily utter detachment. One way or another, the Departing ordinarily know the company they are keeping. And leaving.

Hello Central.

ANTHROPOLOGY

In theology, "anthropology" refers to the sum of a religion's notions of what makes us human.

At the bedside during Long and Last Days, so much of the person you knew may be shed or lost or compromised, or even defiled, that you begin to wonder not only about →accidentals and essences but about root definitions. Ideally, the Departing would exit painlessly, senses intact, with those at the bedside all of one heart--no squabbling, no melodramatic despair, no grasping at straws, no denial of inevitabilities. Indeed, such a kind, genteel departure momentarily suspends all the problematics of being historically human, as if during the Last Days, or the Last Moments of the Last Days, the dying obviates all that has passed for human in the rest of life--the pain, the losses, the uncontrollable desires, the obsessiveness, the relentlessness, the ambition, the fantasizing, the eventual making do.

And where the departure is neither kind nor genteel, neither painless nor alert, and the Departing is barely recognizable or barely there, you may still assume that she deserves to witness us at our best, that he serves as most piercing witness of what we would wish humanity to be known by, every day, all year long. {→Identity}

One might say that it is in the Longest and Last Days that the living reconstitute themselves according to what is most admirably human about humanity. But in that period of reconstitution, do we make ourselves unrecognizable to the Departing? Struggling against a history of personal precedents, trying to be steadily thoughtful, devoted, focused, empathic, responsive, and deeply unselfish, do we make ourselves at once more than we have ever been and less richly complex than we always were?

Strange, how in the Longest and Last Days we may come to question the nub of who we are even as we seek out the hub of what we can be.

ANXIETY

Whether for that diffuse anxiety of losing one's bearings and capacities or for more distinct anxieties associated with specific physical changes, the seriously ill and certainly the Departing are given an "anxiolytic" drug called lorazepam (Ativan). Ativan abets morphine, so the two are usually given together in anticipation of pain and of the anxiety that pain itself can cause.

Being given unanticipated doses of anxiolytics and narcotics can itself make people anxious. What drug are they giving me now? I don't want to be numbed out of my skull and I don't really need more painkillers right now, so if they're giving me Ativan and morphine something awful must be in the works, right?

Ativan is not given to those of us at the bedside who become anxious. What then are the antidotes to our anxieties? To the anxiety that comes of not knowing what to do next, or of being overwhelmed by →checklists and complex regimes of care? To the anxiety that comes of interruptions or interference from busy-bodies, →bounty hunters, →moths. To the anxiety that comes of being in the audible presence of pain, his moans, her screams. Or to the anxiety that comes of not knowing how you are going to manage in the Days After, and the days after that.

The following are anxiolytics (anxiety-reducers):
--People to share the burdens and difficult times at the bedside.
--A sheet of simple instructions for those at the bedside, so they know what to do in stressful or alarming situations {→Acuteness, Aspiration, Tubes, Urgency}
--A good night's →sleep, with dreams.
--An hour's exercise out of doors, running, walking, gardening.
--Fluids (water, water, water, which helps resolve constipation, a more common side-effect of anxiety than diarrhea).
--Taking off your shoes while at the bedside.
--Banning all violent talk shows, shouted newscasts, reality tv.
--Doing art: doodling, sketching, drawing, painting; sharing the making of a collage.
--Reading aloud (but no gruesome murder mysteries or horror stories unless requested).
--Walking the dog (unless the dog is also anxious).
--Learning how to →sit.
--Comfort foods.
→Music (by trial and error: old favorites may not work, and music that works for you may not work for those abed).

You know some others. It will help just to write them down:

APPLES & ORANGES

Death is not an illness. Illnesses are →accidentals, death is of our essence.

People used to be allowed to die of old age, of frailty, even of melancholy. Today, the conditions preceding death have acquired the trappings of illness: not age but Alzheimer's; not frailty but arterial degeneration. A person must die of a known medical cause; it reflects badly on →physicians for anyone to die "of unknown causes," so unknown causes are disappearing. This may be a sign of medical progress or medical hubris.

Cultural and scientific drives to associate the period before death with a disease entity or organ failure have consequences for those at the bedside. They give license to doctors and nurses to interrupt serious conversations for minor tests and monitoring, if not also to press for experimental treatments.

One would think that during the Last Days, at least, you and the Departing could both be free of such interruptions and pressures, but this is rarely the case, whether in hospital or →SNF or even at →home under →hospice care. So long as death is regarded as a disease, there will be problems; so long as mortality is twinned with morbidity, there will be confusions. Am I here at the bedside to help my loved one defend against sepsis or to keep company? Am I here to be a nurse's aide, a medical ethicist, an anaesthetist, or a good friend, a child, a lover, a sister, a brother?

Illness may be used as a metaphor, but that is metaphor ill-used. Pain may be our lot: let theologians and philosophers debate. However, there is something to be said for death, and it may be you who has to say it {→Frankness}. In the Last Days, we are concerned not with sickness, not with illness, not with malady; we are concerned with departure.

Departure has its own rhythms, which should not be disturbed by unnecessary trays of food or the plumping up of pillows. There is a difference between making a person comfortable and guarding against secondary infections, a difference that becomes clearer as Long Days become Last Days--a difference that you may have to insist upon.

It will not be hard to tell the Apples from the Oranges, vigilance from lovingkindness, neediness from necessity, It may take grit to tell others what you and the Departing are about.

ARS MORIENDI, OR THE ART OF DYING

Each spiritual tradition has advice on how to proceed with one's own Last Days, as well as an iconography and choreography of dying. Most traditions also have rituals and texts that encourage one to meditate upon death, sometimes daily.

Less guidance is out there on how to →sit with the Departing during Long and prospectively Last Days. The arts inevitably dramatize the tensions between the living and the dying; novelists and playwrights fix upon battles of wills, shocking revelations, besought confessions, quests for forgiveness, or a fatal hesitation and final stubborn silence on all sides.

Can an artful death be compromised by those at the bedside? Can an artless death be rescued from itself? Should you be a scribe? an archivist? an ombudsman? a mirror?{→Reflection}

It is easier to recognize the artistry of a person's departure than the artistry of those who at the bedside.

Of what does the artistry of the bedside consist? You may consult the manuals of nurses and hospice organizations, the treatises of pastoral counselors, the thick texts on palliative care, all of which are thoughtful and well-meaning, but these have for the most part abandoned the notion of artistry, espousing instead such ideals as compassion, equity, honesty, respectful privacy, and emotional availability. When put into practice in the same room at the same time, these ideals, each worthy and hard-won, are often contentious: equity is not necessarily compatible with compassion; privacy and honesty are not necessarily compatible with each other; availability, stretched thin, can be dishonest. What to do?

The most profound works of art ask questions at the same instant that they heighten contrasts or deepen contexts. They are not smug. They are not *Jeopardy* answers. They are complete but not insular, coherent but neither encyclopedic nor authoritarian. They hope that you will be engaged enough to make more of them, by virtue of your own life, than they are as stand-alones.

So also at the bedside, you are not simply a fall-back or a witness. The longer you are at the bedside, the more likely that you will be called upon to share in the making of an artful death. This will demand compassion, equity, honesty, respect, and emotional availability, but it will also entail a collaboration that is always hard-won, and never smug, and never something you would have known quite how to effect on your own.

ASCITES

Rushing to the bedside, you expect to find a gaunt, sallow figure and instead she is fat, fleshy, and flushed. What's going on? Is all this extra weight good for him? She looks so bloated. Is there a bowel blockage, you've heard these can be fatal. Or maybe he's had so little exercise while eating like normal and a good appetite is a good sign, right? Yet it doesn't seem right for her to be gaining weight and volume at such a pace, maybe it's one aspect of the disease that the doctors didn't bother to mention, or a side-effect of medications--steroids, say.

It's ascites: an accumulation of excess fluids in the peritoneal cavity of the abdomen. The fluids are not inside the abdominal organs or intestines but in that flexible space between them and the membranes lining the abdominal wall. The fluids are transudates (low protein, low molecular weight, clear fluid) or exudates (high protein, with higher molecular weight and much cell debris). Transudates accumulate during heart failure, cirrhosis, or kidney disease. Exudates gather in healthy bodies around a lesion or inflammation; in disease, they gather as a result of cancers and of chemotherapies, which add dead cells to the mix. Diagnostic paracentesis (inserting a →needle through the abdominal wall to sample for transudates or exudates) can become therapeutic when used to withdraw liters of excess fluid, but the fluid will quickly build up again.

Those with massive ascites (as much as 25 liters=55 pounds) may experience shortness of breath due to the weight of the fluid impinging on the diaphragm. Longstanding ascites increases vulnerability to bacterial infections and to portal vein thrombosis. If transudative, ascites can be treated with a low-salt diet and diuretics; if exudative, with paracentesis; in cases of extreme jeopardy, with a shunt. During the Last Days it is left alone and may subside as the body shuts down.

You will how be astonished at how calmly nurses and doctors regard ascites. While the populace spends billions on weight-loss products, while tummy tucks have gained favor when diets fail, and while public health campaigns are waged against an epidemic of obesity, the illusive obesity of ascites is paid never no mind by the medical world. You meanwhile may find yourself hard put to suppress an aesthetic disgust or athletic disquiet at such ungainliness. You may also be disturbed at how difficult it is now to move or →turn the person in bed with all that excess, "sloppy" abdominal weight.

Blame the disease, not the person. Ascites is unrelated to appetite, willpower, or a passion for chocolates.

ASPIRATION

During the Last Days, the Departing begins to breathe with a noisy sucking sound that you suppose must be excruciatingly painful, as if each breath were a battle against being swallowed up by mud or quicksand.

Medical texts assure us that such aspirating is neither painful nor laborious. It is, they assure us, as common near the end as are irregular Cheyne-Stokes respirations in which breathing becomes shallower and slower, to the point of stopping for as long as a minute, succeeded by a number of quick, deep, loudly-drawn breaths. Opening a →window to bring in a breeze, directing a gentle fan toward the bed, elevating the head of the bed, or turning the Departing onto her side may help, but the Cheyne-Stokes respirations can go on for half an hour before more regular breathing resumes.

The clearly audible strangeness of the breathing can frighten children who are visiting the bedside for the first time. At →night, breathing irregularities can be particularly worrisome to those at the bedside, much like sleep apnea.

All who will be at the bedside should know beforehand that the onset of such breathing is no cause for raising an alarm, since it is a typical part of the process of "actively dying" and is not as painful as it seems. Even the moaning that may accompany each breath is simply the sound of air passing over relaxed vocal cords, and not the sound of pain.

An asthmatic, I have my doubts about these reassurances. Could it be that those among the Departing who have suffered through decades of emphysema or asthma may be particularly distressed by aspirated breathing or by Cheyne-Stokes respirations? Certainly it is harder for me in the best of health to listen to labored or interrupted breathing than it is for others who have not experienced the gasping and noisy wheezing of an asthma attack. My body is far too willing to share the forced rhythms of another's struggle for air in an act of all-too-dangerous empathy.

I confess I have delayed writing about this, and I feel reluctant to continue. There is, in addition to aspiration, some probability of dyspnea, physically painful breathing that may, like asthmatic breathing, be exaggerated by panic. Drugs or →music to relieve →anxiety can help here.

ASPIRATION, continued

Listening to the aspirating, the dyspnea, and the Cheyne-Stokes respirations is like listening to a spring-wound clock that is winding down and becoming at once noisier and more unpredictable. It is still telling time, still creating the conditions by which time is told, yet it makes clocktime frighteningly unreliable. So the breathing of the Departing brings you back into time from slow afternoons at the bedside when the hours seemed to lose themselves in opiate daydreams, but it brings you back with a lurch, unsure of what will happen next.

So take a breath of your own. Some deep breaths. Every couple of hours at the bedside, be sure to take some deep breaths. But avoid trying to match your breaths to those of the sleeping aspirating body near you, which goes stutter-step on its way toward a departure you can only hope is as comfortable as they say.

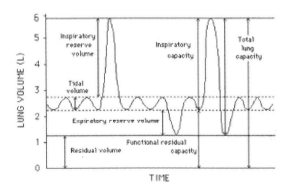

BEDSORES

Those are fortunate who are not confined to bed during the Long Days and Last Days. If they can sit in a chair, walk to the commode or bathroom, stand for a while looking out a →window, they will be better off in all ways. During the Last Weeks, they may well have done all or some of these things, to assert whatever remaining dominion they have over their bodies and their environment.

Being too weak or in too much pain to get out of bed, or paralyzed, or imprisoned by medical equipment, may be as great a blow to one's sense of self as receiving a diagnosis of a terminal illness. To be alive, isn't it to be in motion? To be bedridden for the remainder of one's life seems a cruel rehearsal for death.

Having an adjustable hospital bed at home helps with the sadness of immobility, the feeling that one is no longer free to open the door and run out into the morning. But being bedridden gets old quickly, especially if she had been accustomed just a few months ago to jogging, he to walking the dog each day.

That's the affective soreness of twenty-four hours in bed, day in, day out. The physical sore is the pressure ulcer (decubitis) or bedsore, an area of damaged skin found usually on the shoulder blades, elbows, buttocks, hips, or heels. Bedsores develop when a person is confined to bed for as little as three days, during which pressure from a mattress (yes, it pushes against the body) can cut off circulation, especially when one cannot easily or often change positions. {→Turning.} The friction or shearing from slowly sliding down a mattress can also cause bedsores, as can an ill-fitting bra or rubbing against bed linens grimy from incontinence or sweat.

Alternating-pressure air mattresses have an electromechanical pump that varies the pressure at many points around the mattress to help prevent bedsores. Air-fluidized beds suspend the body on a mattress filled with silicon-coated beads. Memory foam mattresses, which do not push back at the body, may also provide relief.

BEDSORES, continued

If the Departing does contract a bedsore, it can be assessed by its stage:

I. Persistently red (or blue, purple, or ashen) skin that itches or stings and usually feels warm and spongy and sometimes flaky to the touch.

II. An open sore resembling a blister, with the nearby tissue purple or red and superficial (epidermal) or deeper (dermal) skin loss, and beginning to smell.

III. A crater-like wound with damage extending to the tissue below the skin.

IV. A large-scale erosion of tissue, with damage to muscle, bone, joints.

Stages I and II can be managed by cleansing, semipermeable dressings, and dry bed linens. Keep the wound lubricated, the skin around it dry. Use no antiseptics (which injure compromised skin); do apply an antibiotic cream. Stage III requires the removal of dead (necrotic) or infected tissue. Bedsores at Stage IV are sites of lethal infection, but the necessary surgery is rarely performed during the Last Days.

So: pay attention when the seriously ill or Departing complain of an itch or a blister. Soreness about being bedridden, that too must be addressed.

In this regard: the icon that I am using throughout these pages bears reference to the control panel on the arms of electrically adjustable hospital beds. Notice that however one may use the arrows to adjust the bed, the figure has its heels, buttocks, and lower back on the (mattress) surface. These are exactly the places where bedsores begin.

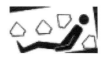

BLACKMAIL

Sometimes it's a joke, sometimes not, and sometimes it's hard to know. Those in their Last Months and Days may ask you to do something you would rather not, or promise to be someone you would rather not be, because you owe them at least this much before they die. Much more, actually, but they're asking only for *this*, and it would mean a great deal to their peace of mind to know that at last you are heading in the right direction. It's only a step or two from this kind of blackmail to a dying curse, which is out of fashion these days and may never have been in fashion except for fairy tales. And already I seem to be shifting in tone from the vicious to the light-hearted, as if it were difficult to be of one mind or mood about deathbed blackmail, since it is at once so anxiously tragic and comically transparent {→*Quid Pro Quo; Quid Pro Quo*, In Reverse}.

One would think, logically, that the blackmail can be operated the other way around, that those at the bedside can threaten to abandon the bedridden if they do not agree to stipulations for a child or spouse or business partner. However, blackmail rarely, and ineffectually, comes from this direction. In fact, during the Last Days the Departing may not mind being left alone.

Blackmail can come in the Last Months from →physicians and surgeons. If the Departing (or you on their behalf) seem too critical of medical or surgical decisions or of religious or ethical stands taken by a doctor or hospital, the doctor may threaten to withdraw or stop the application process for experimental trials. Such blackmail--leaving the Departing in a medical lurch unless the "carping" stops and you all quiet down--is quite effective and not uncommon as a way to keep you from seeking second opinions. This is no joke, although it is unusual for a physician to withdraw entirely, less rare for surgeons (who have more at stake in keeping their success rates high).

The response to blackmail need not be immediate. Give yourself time to assess what is going on. Blackmail works best when you think there's not enough time left to look for other options; it stops working, paradoxically, when there is no time left. Blackmail may begin when the Departing has no other way in which to make a departure decisive and meaningful; it ceases when a larger community of meaning can be invoked.

The bottom line is that we live first for those around us who are living, not for the dead. We honor the wishes of the Departing when their wishes are honorable, and we fulfill our promises to them as best we can in a mutable world. Our lives are not engraved in their stones.

BLANKETS and PILLOWS

It's something you think nothing of: tucking in blankets that have shaken loose; rearranging the pillows. Then it turns out that the pillows are at particular angles beneath the head and neck, below the shoulders, and supporting the back in order to avoid →bedsores or keep mucous out of the way of breathing.

And the blankets and upper sheets are laid out in an obviously expert if mysterious way that makes it easier to →turn a person or to change the bed. You didn't know you had to have special training just to move a pillow or straighten the covers, and you throw up your hands in despair. How can you be of any help at the bedside if the simplest things require years of training?

What's with the sheets and blankets, anyway? The Departing is picking at them, determinedly picking at them, as if they are too thin and old and are shedding lint. Can't the Departing afford a new set of sheets, a sturdier blanket, a better coverlet?

Then it turns out that the concerted picking is a neuromuscular (or neurocognitive and hallucinatory) sign of the Last Days {→Floccillation}, and there's nothing wrong with the sheets or blankets. Indeed, new sheets unless extremely soft, and very expensive, would be too rough on vulnerable skin.

In addition, the internal thermostat of the seriously ill is going to fluctuate, sometimes wildly, and the blanket will be tossed off or pulled up at the oddest intervals, so how can you know when to help with something ostensibly so simple as covers?

Pillows under the head will be pummeled or endlessly plumped, shoved around or out of the way because of . . . earache, or wanting to hear? Drool on the pillow slips? Migraines?

Ask the nurses or hired →caregivers to let you in on their bed-linen skills and the use of pull sheets. Ask respectfully, for they are proud of how they can manage even the most ungainly, obstreperous, or pained of bodies.

You might also consider your frustration with blankets and pillows as an element of a larger perplexity that we all face. Are we at the bedside in anticipation only of special moments of tender remembrance, deep communion, direct confession? Or because this is where we belong? Or because there is a certain honor to being now in the presence of the Departing, however humdrum the days, however unsettling our own uncertainties about "being in the way." Or because, blankets and pillows aside, there are other conversations to be had, other comforts to be taken, other cares to be addressed?

BLOOD

Five things about blood:

1. Not all illnesses or departures are bloody. In many cases the Departing will be presentable even to the most squeamish. Indeed, the opposite aspect may be more shocking: loss of color in the cheeks and lips, loss of circulation to the hands.

2. Some relationships are stronger than blood. Blood kin may be neither the most welcome nor most understanding nor most compassionate at the bedside. Whatever "blood lines" establish, they do not ground every friendship, every love. Although our hospitals, nursing homes, and courts seem to honor spouses and kin above all others, the Long and Last Days should not be surrounded by a moat of blood. Near the end, the Departing may have more need of a →friend or a current lover than of a relative with whom she grew up or a parent from whom he has been estranged. This is hard to grasp, harder to accept with equanimity. {→Brothers and Sisters; Mothers and Fathers; Wives, Husbands, and Lovers}

3. Blood transfusions sometime help as a way to help the seriously ill and Departing remain alert and to feel, for a while, independent. →Hospice practice rarely permits transfusions, but often a good argument can be made in favor of transfusion as a significantly complementary means for pain relief.

4. In the Last Days, blood may not be something to worry about, however dramatic it may appear. Now that departure is in sight, symptoms lose their urgency and diagnosis is less important. Bloody stools, bloody urine, bloody sputum will be taken by medical staff more casually than one might think they should be taken, or would ordinarily be taken. Blood will no longer be drawn. Blood pressure will decline.

5. Red is an awkward color to have at the bedside. The deep purplish-red of certain roses, for example, resembles too closely the bruises on the arms and wrists of the seriously ill and Departing who have had IVs stuck in them time and again, with leakages and swelling. Nightgown red may seem too obvious an attempt to mask the probability of →bedsores. Dark red lipstick, red fingernail polish, or rouge on dying women looks garish, lurid, nightmarish. And most reds do not fare well under institutional fluorescent lights.

. . . Oh, a sixth thing about blood:

6. Blood banks always need it.

BOUNTY HUNTERS

Caution: Some come to the bedside during the Last Days because they have a quota of souls to rescue--from sin, from unhappiness, from injustice, from despair, from death. They are on a personal mission, on behalf of no church, temple, or spiritual practice. They build up merit and reputation as they move from one hospital floor to another, but their interests lie more with the act of rescue than with the heart or mind of the Departing. They come not to listen but persuade, by subtle threat, by sweetness, or wheedling. They are not easily turned away. They know what it is to be denied access, but five years ago they met the Departing at a bus stop and now it's time for a long talk; or last week in the market they were chatting with a friend of a friend who mentioned that it might be nice to stop in before it was too late, which reminded them of a chance encounter in which, months and months before, the Departing had wondered about Heaven, or whether saints were better known for their martyrdoms than their sense of justice. Bounty Hunters have answers, in the form of proverbs, maxims, or ionizing beams. On the surface they do not appear to be crazed or crackpot, but they are insistent and temperamental-- and oblivious to crowds or the pressure of events. They have to see the Departing: it's a matter of life and death. They know how to insinuate themselves into a situation, bringing a special pillow, aloe juice, wheat grass, a fine soap, so that they seem to be well-meaning. Their eyes, like those of all hunters, are intense. They are acutely sensitive to being slighted or ignored, which they frame in terms of unfairness, injustice, ignorance: if these others who are not family members can visit with the Departing, why not me? How dare you presume to choose the company for the Departing in these Last Days? And just how do you know these are the Last Days? Haven't you given up too soon? {→Have You Thought Of...?} Have you contacted this clinic in Mexico? There's an amazing healer in Brazil who will fly in for special cases. Are you doing all you can do? I have connections, it's possible that she doesn't have to die, that he can get well, and what are you afraid of? Bounty hunters are good at making you feel guilty, inadequate, stingy, uncaring. They know how to make you doubt yourself. They have come to collect on a forgotten promise or an imagined debt, and it's hard to tell whether their claims are oddly true, half-true, cock-eyed, or an elaborate fabrication. They make you feel as if you never really knew the Departing, as if they had been living a parallel life with strange people plugged into networks with arcane knowledge of foreign clinics, jungle herbs, high-altitude therapeutic modalities, hyperbaric oxygen chambers, and

BOUNTY HUNTERS, continued, unfortunately

who are you to say there isn't something to it and worth a try now that there are few other prospects? Bounty Hunters love being the last resorts, they have trained for these moments and are armed to the teeth with URLs, unlisted telephone numbers, rice paper brochures, apocryphal books, secrets that have been suppressed by the military-industrial-medical establishment because if they got out, everyone would live long, in health and in peace, and where would billionaire investors make their profits? The Departing has been misdiagnosed by doctors more concerned about the rising cost of malpractice insurance than about their patients, and people rise from their deathbeds more often than you know. The statistics on wrongful deaths are alarming. Here, I'll show you. Just let me in {→Gatekeeping}. Let me in. Let me in.

In this regard: One might think of bounty hunters as another kind of bedsore.

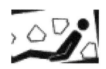

BREASTBONE, or STERNUM

From first to last, touch is elemental to your presence at the bedside. But illnesses with high fevers, or breakthrough pain, make people hypersensitive to the least touch. And then there are the IV insertion points, heart monitor leads, chapped lips, pressure wraps on the legs, pillows placed to prevent clotting and →bedsores, so where *can* you lay a finger?

One hand and forearm are usually free, so holding hands is possible so long as you avoid any bruises on the back of the hand from awkwardly-placed IV →needles. The top of the wrist is also often bruised, and the soft skin of the underwrist can be ticklish, so you must be cautious, especially since the shrinking circumference of the wrist becomes iconic for those who have been watching themselves dwindle {→Diminishing}.

The safest, finest place to touch is most often the top of the breastbone, or sternum, that flat bone at the middle of the ribcage, on the chest between the breasts. Hospice nurses and veteran caregivers know to place a palm gently on the breastbone and talk quietly or not at all; in moments, those who have been restless, fretful, or moaning will calm down.

Stand to either side of the bed and slowly, gently place an open dry palm flat on the breastbone, over the bedclothes, pajamas, or gown. You will feel, *know*, that contact has been made, that your presence has been registered and appreciated. If your own breathing is relaxed, you may be able to feel the person's breathing also relax with your touch.

You are not pushing at the chest like someone practicing resuscitation. You are not doing massage. The steady warmth and lightness of your palm on the breastbone for two, maybe three minutes is all that's needed.

You may want to do this every so often throughout the day, or an anxious night. The power of this touch lies in its directness and simplicity. It is so powerful that five or six minutes of palm to breastbone could feel oppressive to both of you.

In some rare diseases and after some surgeries, you should not try to place a palm on the breastbone. In that case (I have seen it work), place your flat palm in the air an inch or two above the breastbone and let it hover there, quietly.

Try it.

BROTHERS and SISTERS

When it comes to brothers and sisters, prospects of life are often stronger than probabilities of death. Bone marrow or kidney transplants seem to bring brothers and sisters closer together than does the deathbed, which asks for little sacrifice from the living except for time and patience. It's easier, isn't it (because more dramatic and more publicly rewarding) to offer to share a physical part of oneself--blood, marrow, a kidney, even a retina--than to sit at the bedside for hours and endure the presence of someone you are supposed to love but from whom you have been estranged for years. →Blood is not all.

Cruel. Cynical. There must be siblings galore who are tight, who see each other every day or speak warmly with each other every week throughout their lives. These will know what to do for each other during the Long and Last Days and, unless fussbudgets or blowhards, they will do it well.

As for other brothers and sisters who have led lives emotionally or physically distant, divided by geography, religion, politics, and/or style, it would be foolish to claim that grave illnesses and departures always effect reconciliations. Yet the pressure for this to happen is enormous and comes from all directions, →mothers and fathers, distant relatives, friends. The Departing herself may want her deathbed to be the setting for treaties of non-aggression among siblings, or pacts between ancient adversaries. When will a childhood grudge be remitted, a grievance dismissed, if not now? What brother wants to go to the grave with a festering wound? What sister wants to send another off to the cemetery with a cutting remark?

But we are not all philosophical at the end. Whether for reasons of rivalry, distrust, or stern recrimination, some brothers and sisters may be no better for each other in the Long and Last Days than they were in the prior decades. Issues of birth order and privilege, of betrayal or denial, may resurface regardless of crisis and finality. Or there may be a superficial restraint in the interests of being pleasant, a holding back that becomes, in the Days After, a bequest of bitterness.

For younger siblings, Long and Last Days can seem particularly troubling because these feel premonitory, as in "this is how I also will go," or "this is not how I intend to die," so a tension arises. For older siblings, they may say to themselves, I should have gone first, or I should have done a better job of looking after the Departing, so it would not have come to this.

Who sells no-fault insurance for brothers and sisters?

BUYING TIME

For whom? From whom?

Such an odd turn of phrase, "buying time." As if dying were part of a commercial transaction. As if you could bank time like blood and draw it out when needed. As if there were lending institutions for second mortgages on life.

During the Long Days and Last Months, "buying time" makes it possible to search out experimental treatments or confirm a prognosis; during the →Last Days, buying time makes it possible for some farewells to be made in person. During the →Last Months and Weeks, the Departing may have the time and alertness to sign the necessary legal documents. During the Last Days, you may wish to think that you can "buy time" for the Departing with special care or good company; but really you have little purchase on the time of death once it is so close.

Buying time is a way to "delay the inevitable." Another odd turn of phrase, usually modified by just or only: we're just delaying the inevitable, you're only delaying the inevitable. Last Days do imply an irreversibility that makes the buying of time seem, if not foolish, futile. Hoping against hope.

Another odd turn of phrase, that. "Hoping against hope." Is it that one cannot say that one hopes the Departing departs sooner rather than later, with less days of pain or confusion?

Or is the thought of the departure so intimidating that you yourself would rather buy a little more time, as if you were buying vowels at the Wheel of Fortune to keep on spinning.

On whose behalf are you looking to buy time? Is there something else for the Departing to do, a bucket list (as in the 2007 film with Morgan Freeman and Jack Nicholson) of exotic destinations, reparations, skydiving? Skydiving?

And exactly how does your time coincide with the time you say you want to buy for the Departing, when the departure is accompanied by Alzheimer's, or the silence of end-stage Parkinson's, or the →pain of cancer in the bone?

Every year news articles appear on how much a human body is worth. The amount varies from $4.50 for the body as a collection of minerals and membranes, $45,000,000 for the body as a bank for organs, blood, DNA, and bone marrow. A departure dedicated to →organ transfers is actually buying time: for others.

Do not sell departures short.

CALENDARS

Walls don't always have ears, as much as you might want that to be so, dashing from the bedside to the bathroom or kitchen. Walls do have openings: doors, →windows, air vents, calendars. That's right: calendars. Although wall calendars have become icons of deadlines and closure, calendars more often open out than turn in upon themselves.

I am thinking both of the photographs or paintings above the fold and of the numbered day-squares below. Calendar images, thankfully, are never of hospital bedtables festooned with ointments and spit basins, never of institutional corridors or aluminum walkers. Jeffrey Kittay, writing about those with the most limited abilities to share their sensations and make their wishes known, suggests that even two-dimensional images on hallway walls can become a kind of inevitable *trompe l'oeil*, leading the eye and mind toward believing in what is not immediately here. That is one of the stranger powers of art, to effect presence while insisting on other places, different times.

The day-squares, too, open upon prospect. Everyone in the room is here now, on this day with the empty square, so in point of fact the square is neither empty nor putative. Filling in the daily squares with the names of visitors, procedures, future appointments, reminders and phone numbers, that is a good thing, better than the standard holidays posted from month to month, since the filling-in is evidence of lively presence and a prompt toward context.

You might also attach quotations from recent letters or snippets from postcards, but the ambition of such filling-in is not fullness, it is motion, the dynamic relation of place and time. In bed or beside it, you have *all* been doing things, awake or half-conscious, through time; let no one dismiss your hours and days as wasted or lost.

Nor need you →X out the days as each one passes, as if histories could be obliterated. Indeed, it will prove invaluable to the maintenance of a medical →history and profile if you keep the past months attached as you fold back one image to find the next, building up behind the current month a bulwark of assurances: you have *all* been here, there's more to come.

I might avoid calendars whose artwork is too cute, gauzy, fussy, or pointedly polemic (e.g., teddy bears posed at tea tables or animal species in danger of extinction), but matters of taste should be left to the ill and Departing. In any case, choose a calendar with large bold squares that can be seen distinctly from a distance.

CALENDARS, continued

The most alert of patients and steadfast of caregivers may lose track of time after too many days in hospital or a →skilled nursing facility, as medical routines supplant one's typical markers of morning, noon,→ night, another day. Nurses each morning at shift change may write the new day and date on a wallboard in front of each bed, but a calendar situates everyone within the longer run of events, and opens always toward places and beings beyond the walls.

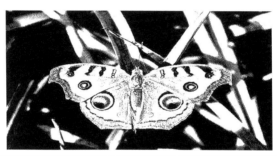

what	has	been	going	on	?	What
have	you	been	doing	here	?	Whose
birth	day	is	it?	Who	is	on
her	way	here?	Can	I	draw	or
paint	in	this	square	?		

CAREGIVERS--HIRING

Should →Mutual Peril or other circumstances dictate and finances permit, you may be charged with helping to find, hire, and sometimes discharge private caregivers.

Caregivers may be found by hospital or private →Case Managers; through home care →agencies; through social workers or eldercare specialists; online through Craig's List or at websites established by caregivers; by recommendation from friends, neighbors, visiting nurses, or physicians. However you find them, they must be interviewed for compatibility with the patient and the circle of care {→Caregivers--Interviewing}.

If a prospective caregiver has given a favorable impression through her (rarely, his) c.v. and personal interview, you will want to ask for and contact two references, then institute a background check, which can be done by paying an online service that assures you of no criminal record, no aliases, no serious driving violations, and no outstanding warrants anywhere in the nation. You may also want proof of being drug-free. Agencies have already screened caregivers for criminal records, valid driver's license and, usually, for drugs. You can ask for the results of these screenings and a copy of the license. Or you can trust your instincts.

Most agencies have bonded their caregivers, which means that they have a policy with a bonding company that compensates for employee theft and destruction of property. If you hire through an agency, bonding would seem to protect you against theft and property damage, but homeowner's or renter's insurance policies and the guarantees behind most credit cards already cover this, and in any case a full formal criminal investigation must be concluded before compensation kicks in. (Self-employed caregivers can pay to bond themselves, but this is expensive, as is the bonding of a set of caregivers by a household that's hired them privately.)

Agencies also pay all the taxes for caregivers. This is particularly important if you are hiring full-time (live-in, twenty-four-hour) caregivers: if you hire privately and pay any caregiver over $1400 per calendar year (a number the IRS may change), then you must file payroll taxes for each with regard to Social Security, Medicare, federal and state unemployment and disability insurance, and advance payment of earned income credit for eligible employees. You would also have to report wages on a quarterly basis and pay quarterly state unemployment taxes. You may not have to do income tax withholding, but by law you must furnish employee(s) with a Form W-2 no later than January 31 of the following year. You cannot avoid these taxes by hiring a caregiver as an independent contractor. On this and more, consult www.caregiver.com/articles/general/caregivers_and_taxes.htm

Live-in caregivers ordinarily get both room and board in exchange for a daily rate of pay that is about half the cost of hiring at an hourly rate for 24 hours. But they too must be allowed days off, so if round-the-clock care is imperative, you will need to hire a second caregiver for respite. If hiring privately, you will also want to have at hand a neighbor or friend who can be called upon in emergencies to stay overnight.

Other than long-term care insurance policies, no insurance in the United States pays for caregivers.

This is reprehensible. As the philosopher Eva Kittay has argued in *Love's Labor* (1999), the human condition is grounded in caregiving. At birth, in early childhood, during injury or illness, and on the approach of death, each of us is dependent on other human beings, a circle of care that makes us possible. That circle of care almost always expands beyond kin and is elemental not only to our survival but to a longterm sense of well-being that enables us in all else we do.

We should therefore honor those "strangers" who tend to us, whether as nannies or in pre-schools, as orderlies and aides in hospital wards or nursing facilities, or at the bedside at home. Instead, we pay them little, as if they were "unskilled," and neither personally nor politically set aside anything for their vital, necessary presence. And they will be necessary, for almost everyone of us, at some time down the line.

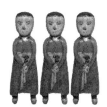

CAREGIVERS--INTERVIEWING {also: Agencies}

Hiring caregivers entails interviews.

Your questions for caregivers will be determined, of course, by the personality as well as the illness and status of the person to be cared for. (Is she bedridden or likely to be out and about every day? Is he incapacitated in mind or senses, or alert? Does she require hands-on toileting and bathing, or is she mostly in need of a companion on the watch for falls, chills, memory lapses? Does he tend to be mute--did he keep to himself even when well?--or is he highly sociable and hungry for conversation? Is she in great pain?)

Here are some questions to consider asking during interviews:

Experience:
How long have you been a caregiver?
What sort of clients have you worked with?
    elderly? bedridden? paraplegics? diabetics?
    [fill in the blanks:]_____   _____
Have you worked in
    →skilled nursing or board-and-care establishments?
    Alzheimer's units? Mostly at private homes?
Do you prefer to work with people of the same
    gender? faith? ethnicity?

Skills:
Have you worked with
    slide boards? collapsible wheelchairs? Hoyer lifts?
How are you at helping people transfer from
    bed to wheelchair or bath chair?
    into and out of a car?
Have you emptied urine or ostomy bags?
Are you comfortable with all that is required for
    diapering? toileting? bathing? dressing?

Legal/economic issues:
Are you a legal guardian for anyone?
Are you in bankruptcy proceedings?
Do you have a US passport or green card?

Habits and diet:
Do you smoke?
Do you drink beer/wine/liquor?
Are you a vegan? A vegetarian? A diabetic?
    on a low-cholesterol, low-salt, &/or low-fat diet?
Are you a good cook? What are your specialties? {→Food}

Health and Strength:
Are you healthy?
Do you have any back or neck problems?
Any arthritis? Angina? Problems bending or lifting?
Can you push a wheelchair for half a mile?
Are you a walker? A jogger?
Do you enjoy the out-of-doors?

Transportation and Driving:
How far away do you live? Ordinarily, how would you get here?
Do you have a current valid state driver's license?
Would you mind driving a person to doctor's appointments,
    shopping, a movie or a museum, a park?
Is your car in good shape for such excursions?
    Does it have bucket seats? Two doors or four?
    (Bucket seats are incommodious for the weak and elderly;
    two-door cars make transporting a wheelchair more difficult.)

Communication and education:
What languages do you speak?
Do you have any training or certificates in
    first aid? CPR? nursing?
How far did you get in school?
Do you have a working cell phone? Do you text or tweet?
Do you get e-mail? Do you go online daily?

Ask also about interests and hobbies and try to determine
whether a caregiver will be a quiet or noisy companion,
introspective or outgoing, active or passive.

Emergencies:
To whom do you yourself turn in an emergency?
Have you ever called 911 for yourself or for a client?
    If so, what was your experience?
Do you know what a →DNR is?
Do you know about Advance →Directives?

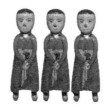

CAREGIVING, CARETAKING

Odd, that these two compounds should mean the same thing. What is it about Long Days and Last Days that makes giving equivalent to taking?

Is it the absence of possessiveness? Would that it were. More often than you might think, the long-term looking-after of a person leads, near departure, to assertions of rights to the attention of the Departing, or to being honored and rewarded for loyalty, or to a fierce protectiveness that gets in the way of attempts at reconciliation among those at the bedside.
{→Gatekeeping}

Is it that the caution of "taking care" elides into the selflessness of "giving care" as a person enters the Last Days? Perhaps, although few are the caretakers who near the end can throw caution to the winds in the interests of an exuberant grand finale, and so caregivers may end up being the most →fatigued and →depressed, sulky or balky of people at the bedside.

Is it that a caretaker is understood as a maintenance worker while a caregiver is thought to intervene at critical moments, but in the Last Days the crisis is constant and, therefore, by definition, fades into maintenance, so that the giving and taking have at last the same ambitions? Yes it is.

At the bedside you cannot avoid being both, hoping for the even keel of caretaking, which is (admit it) at once a tedium and a great relief, and responding as need be to moments of breakthrough →pain or dissociation, which are (admit it) at once a horror and a great reward (it was worth coming, since I could be of help).

We have adages about giving and taking that make the two reciprocal if not identical. Charity, teaching, deep talk all seem to share a notion of the reciprocity of giving and taking, of caring. The caring is important.

What you must guard against is caregiving as an act of rationing, caretaking as a constrictive, debilitating wariness. The Departing need pass through no further narrows than those already on the map before you came.

Nor need you.

CASCADES

Miles in and up through wilderness, you might have hiked to stand beside one of these or eat lunch in their spray.

In mathematical and medical terms, a cascade is a series of connected, branching events that have their own momentum, usually swift and somewhat unpredictable because of the different possible routes and ramifications.

Last Days are fraught with cascades, as one bodily system after another fails. It's not entirely predictable--as with thunderous waterfall--where the spray will go, how the streams will dash against the rocks . . . when the legs or eyes or heart will go. A cascade is swift but half-random, a randomness we seek out in the High Sierras but not at the bedside.

The cascades of the Last Days are inaudible, sometimes invisible. They are fearsome because they catch you unaware, their rhythms strangely impersonal, as if proceeding despite outward signs of good health and fine spirits. The cascade, whatever its origins, appears to be a force of its own.

To a casual observer, the departure may seem deliberate, while on the inside of the body all hell has broken loose.

You leave for the evening, confident that these are not the →Last Hours, since the Departing has a bloom in her cheeks and a strong voice, then you get a call at 11:30 that it's all over, she's gone, there was nothing to be done. Cascade.

One moment you are talking with the Departing about world events and what should be done about poverty or hunger, the next moment there is silence or hard breathing and a very low pulse. Cascade.

Cascades occur because . . . no, they do not occur because of any one thing. The nature of a cascade is confluence. As conception is an extraordinary confluence, so is death. Much of life is dedicated to building dams and conduits against complexity, making forces predictable and events manageable. During the Long Days, everyone is still building dams, repairing conduits. During the Last Days, you try to make yourself comfortable with the thought that at least you know that these are the Last Days. Behind the scenes, however, like mountain water melting under glaciers, there are streams descending toward powerful if indeterminate confluences. Cascade.

Since most death comes by unseen, unheard cascade, dying is always, if predictably, →sudden.

CASE MANAGEMENT

During the Long Days, you may want or need to help with so much that you can be overwhelmed. Scheduling appointments with doctors and therapists, or with radiology units and imaging centers. Ordering, refilling, and administering drugs, ointments, eye drops at different times of day. Assisting with injections, urine collections, suppositories, baths. Emptying spit buckets, ostomy bags. Replacing dressings, applying lotions. Preparing meals that follow detailed but contradictory dietary guidelines. Searching medical texts to make sense of what a doctor said. Looking online for experimental trials. Assembling evidence for second opinions or writing insurance appeals.

You *can* do all of this, and the shopping, the laundry, the mending, the watering of flowers, feeding of pets, calling in of plumbers or computer techs. You can also answer phones and e-mails, welcome guests, check out books or DVDs from the library, and all else that amounts to what authorities call the Activities of Daily Living (ADLs). But how are you bearing up?

Then there will be periods when you are at a hospital bedside. This may feel like a respite from the ADLs noted above, but still you will want to keep track of shifting diagnoses or treatments, and you will need to wait to catch the hospitalist or specialist to get questions answered, lab results explained. You may need to ask for a new room if the roommate is so noisy (coughing, hacking, moaning, screaming) that your loved one cannot get any sleep. You may need to watch for errors in the meals sent up by the kitchen. You *can* do all this, chasing down doctors, gatekeeping, companionship, but how are you bearing up?

Prior to discharge, it may devolve upon you to find, visit, and select an acceptable →skilled nursing facility, assisted living complex, or board-and-care. You may have to help decide whether it's best for the ill or Departing to go →home and if so, whether to hire →caregivers, and if so, whether they should be live-in or hourly, Certified Nursing Assistants or Licensed Vocational →Nurses or non-credentialed but experienced companions? And what about a wheelchair--which kind is available, which is best? What are hi-lo beds? What's a slideboard? a Hoyer lift? {→Doodads.}

Or maybe it's time to contract with a →hospice that will take care of all medical issues. How choose between the competing hospice groups, and how do you know what to ask them?

Yes, you *can* figure this all out, slog through everything without collapsing, but for how long? Everyone in the circle of care may also be feeling overwhelmed, especially when family live out of town. You may be embarrassed to admit that you need help, but when you find that you've put your own life on hold for so long that you resent the demands at the bedside, yet feel guilty for that resentment and oppressed by that guilt, it is more than time to seek outside help.

Here's where private case (or care) managers come in. They are costly; no insurance other than some long-term-care policies pay for their services. But they take in hand as much of the above as you (all of you) would like: transitions from hospital to home or elsewhere; caregiver or companion hiring and supervision; prescriptions; diet; scheduling; transport; attendance at doctor's offices, ERs, hospital bedsides, surgery recovery units, ICUs. They can act as medical translators among physicians, nurses, family, lovers, friends, and even insurance providers. They maintain updated medical histories and lists of meds and implanted devices. They check on a client's mental, emotional, and physical status and quality of ongoing care. They can bring in ombudsmen, file complaints, seek out alternative programs or treatments, find doctors for second opinions. They are advocates for their client in all situations, articulating and defending a client's interests, asking the appropriate questions, compiling the records. {→History, Part II}

They may also advise on necessary medico-legal documents, but should not be signatories to or beneficiaries of wills and never should have power of attorney or guardianship.

To be nationally certified as a case manager, one must have started with an MD, a nursing degree (RN or LVN), or social work (MSW), then passed a specific curriculum. Most case managers will have a medical or social work background and be on staff at hospitals or →SNFs. There is however no state or federal licensure of case managers, so anyone (like me) can set up a private case management business. Ask for references, including one from a physician.

The more isolated is the seriously ill or Departing from a circle of care, the more you may need to entertain the prospect of hiring a case manager. If finances make this possible.

Somewhat less expensive is concierge care, where several neighbors in similar jeopardy enlist a "concierge" who brings to bear many free services or low-cost community resources.

In any case, the person ailing or abed must agree to such help.

CATHETERS

Definition: A flexible →tube for insertion into a body cavity, duct, or vessel to allow the passage or drainage of fluids.

Most commonly, catheters are inserted into the urethra under local anaesthetic. They are meant to keep the flow of urine from requiring continual attention when a person is temporarily or permanently incontinent. Temporarily: while undergoing surgery, suffering a bladder infection, or as a side-effect of stiff doses of nasal decongestants, alpha blockers, anti-depressants, antihistamines, calcium channel blockers. Permanently: from paralysis, injury, or stroke; from prostate or bowel surgery.

Ostomy patients also use catheters, often permanently, to drain urine, sometimes fecal matter, sometimes both. In the U.S. there are at least a million people who have had colostomies, ileostomies, or urostomies and are leading lives otherwise unremarkable--or remarkable, as the case may be.

→Sitting at the bedside of someone with a catheter, you may notice a tube leading out from under the covers to a drainage bag hooked to the bed. In hospitals, the urine accumulating in the bag will be measured and emptied at regular intervals. At home, there will rarely be a need to measure. {→Dialysis.}

It's up to you whether you want to use gloves when emptying the catheter bag. {→Hands and Gloves.} Some people can empty their own catheter bags, and some can even change out their own catheters. Permanent (in-dwelling) catheters should be changed at least once a month and often need to be flushed with a solution of acetic acid in order to prevent the growth of bacteria and development of Urinary Tract Infections (UTIs), which can affect men as well as women, causing pain, fever, night sweats, fatigue, and serious mental confusion that itself may be confused with symptoms of other infections.

For travel, there are smaller bags with shorter tubing, so that a person can fit the bag inside a dress or trousers and it won't get in the way of greater mobility.

I continue to be impressed at how quickly those at the bedside learn to accept and work with catheter tubes and bags, and how the inevitable daily conversations about the color, clarity, and flow of urine gradually introduce even the most reticent to close medical observation. You could say that catheter bags, which may be a permanent presence during the Long Days through to the Last, are like Yield signs on highways: cautions of entrance and exit, of slowing down, of looking ahead for traffic and intersections, for crossroads and fellow travelers.

CATS, DOGS, AND PARROTS

Cats and dogs often sense the Last Days of their owners and will come to lie quietly with them, for hours. Their company reduces the felt levels of →pain and restores calm.

Cats and dogs *can* cause problems, and not just their dander or fleas. During an illness or Departure, they may be fiercely protective, hissing or barking at visitors. They may refuse to eat. They may stop using the litter box or refuse to go outside. They may resist flea treatments or their own medicines.

Such behavior may be a sign of mourning. Animals who live with us →grieve with us and for us. When you come to sit at the bedside of someone who has a dog, cat, or parrot that has been with the person for years, you are the outsider and must, initially, defer to them. They may be more important to the Departing than anything else, any*one* else, in this life.

With that in mind, you may need to coax the pets to eat, take medicines, return to the litter box or yard; the Departing will be more anxious on their behalf than on yours. The dying do not forget their closest friends.

If the departure is taking place in a hospital or →SNF, and if rules permit, bring the Departing's dog or parrot or cat to the room. More and more commonly, pet visits are being allowed, and companion dogs (with their trainers) may rove the halls.

But this happens too, in the Last Days: a dog or cat will vanish, and the Departing will be far more concerned about that disappearance than about his or her own departure.

Some pets, nervous or completely dependent on the Departing, do freak out. In this case, you will need the help of a veterinarian or animal trainer.

After the Departing has gone, dogs and particularly parrots (who are monogamous and bond for life, either with a mate or, in lieu of a mate, with the human who cares for them) have been known to waste away and die from loss and grief. Aside from tortoises, parrots are the longest-lived of common pets and can live for eighty (human) years, so those that do not die from grief may survive for a long time. Although →wills often make provisions for their care by another family member or a bird sanctuary, parrots are not likely to bond with a subsequent owner. Dogs can recover more quickly.

At the bedside, observe the pets. You may learn more from them about the physical and emotional status of the ill and the Departing than from a doctor, nurse, or caregiver.

CELL (mobile) PHONES

Picture the Departing on a cell phone during her Last Minutes, with his →Last Breaths. Or one of those wireless Bluetooth sets with a swash of metal clipped to the ear and talking straight ahead as if delusional. What a different context for →Last Words.

The etiquette of the Last Days with regard to cell phones is changing rapidly as emergency rooms, hospitals, and nursing facilities find it impossible to enforce bans on cell phones in waiting rooms, hallways, or at bedsides.

A few wealthy souls during the 1800s did have their coffins wired for telegraph or telephone service, lest they woke from what had only been a coma to find themselves buried (alive). Before the electroencephalograph and other diagnostic equipment, it was much harder to tell whether someone was fully dead or in a kind of limbo, and the invention of ether and chloroform had complicated matters. Thus the patenting of coffins with wires and bells to ring from within and below.

The constant use of mobile devices, whether by the Departing or among those at the bedside, is not unlike that of encoffined wires: communication at all cost. Some now are probably being buried with a Bluetooth receiver at one ear and holding a cell phone, fully charged.

For 19th-century mediums conducting seances, the idea of communicating with the Other Side was no more farfetched than communicating by telegraph or cable from one side of the Earth to the other, and certainly no more farfetched than communicating by wireless telegraph (that is, radio) from Earth to the planets.

Cell phones are magical in that way: they further the illusion of being endlessly and perfectly in touch, anywhere. Unlike land lines, cell phones do not tie you to a specific site; you can float between places, hover between personalities.

But who do you think you are to be on your cell phone at the bedside of the Departing? What rudeness to allow the outside world to intrude upon these Last Days? Of course, the call might not be for you; it might be for the person who is doing all the heavy lifting called departure.

The next →generations will hardly be alone at death.

CHECKLISTS

Checklists can be helpful so long as they do not become proxies for your full presence at the bedside. They can be calming in times of confusion, give the distracted a sense of direction, and help keep priorities straight. Herewith three brief checklists:

Checklist for Long Days and Last Months:
Have these been completed? Do you know where they are?

Wills and →Directives
- ☐ Advance Health Care Directive, or
- ☐ Living Will and/or
- ☐ Durable →Power of Attorney for Health Care
- ☐ Will and codicils, notarized
- ☐ Living (or other) Trusts, with lawyers' names, contacts

Inventories
- ☐ Of assets, property, with photos or videos
- ☐ Warranties and proofs of purchase

Medical information {→History, Part II}
- ☐ Medical records (hospitals, nursing or rehab facilities)
- ☐ Physician & pharmacy names, contact information
- ☐ List of current →medications and dietary supplements
- ☐ Home care agencies, with contact information

Tax records
- ☐ Current receipts, checkbooks, credit card statements
- ☐ Past three years' tax filings
- ☐ →Social Security number, birthdate and place

Passwords (and numbers for)
- ☐ bank accounts (including ATM cards) {→Money}
- ☐ credit and debit cards
- ☐ stocks, bonds, annuities
- ☐ online / automatic billing accounts
- ☐ cloud archives, e-security, networks

→Keys to
- ☐ safe deposit boxes, home safes, lockboxes
- ☐ cars, trucks, golf carts, RVs, ATVs, boats, bikes
- ☐ house(s) or apartments, including cottages, rental units
- ☐ storage units or pods, sheds, greenhouses

Contact List: family, friends to keep apprised

Checklist for the Last Weeks/Days

Each day/shift should attend to:

Comfort

- ☐ pain?
- ☐ constipation/diarrhea? {→Shit Happens}
- ☐ fever? shivers? sensitivities?{→Hot and Cold)
- ☐ hunger or →thirst?

Environment, adjusted for

- ☐ room temp and humidity?
- ☐ →lighting?

→Medications

- ☐ changes in prescriptions or supplements?
- ☐ new prescriptions or refills needed?

Dressings & →Tubes

- ☐ any to be changed or flushed?
- ☐ enough supplies on hand?

Messages: (update the Contact List)

- ☐ →cell phone or telephone?
- ☐ mail? e-mail? text messages?

Hygiene

- ☐ mouth care?
- ☐ skin care? Always check for →bedsores
- ☐ hands/→nails?
- ☐ →hair?
- ☐ genitals, perineal, and anal area

→Food & Drink:

- ☐ any requests? something to add to the shopping list?
- ☐ what's on hand (is anything going bad in the refrigerator)?

Visits or Visitors Scheduled: {→Gatekeeping}

- ☐ →physicians or visiting nurses?
- ☐ aides or volunteers?
- ☐ family or →friends?

Media: {→Entertainment}

- ☐ →music (and headphones)?
- ☐ books or magazines?
- ☐ tv guide, videos or dvds?

→Laundry to do?:

Checklist for the Days After

Calls and Notifications to make. *Asterisks indicate when you may need a separate→Death Certificate.

- ☐ At death, hospice MD, or GP, who notifies the coroner.
- ☐ Funeral home, burial society, organ donor facility
- ☐ Family attorney*
- ☐ Family & friends--from list compiled in Last Months
- ☐ Local newspapers / trade journals for →obituaries

Medical:

- ☐ Hospice and other →Nurses (thank-you cards)
- ☐ Home Health →Agencies / Grooming/ Massage

Governmental

- ☐ →Social Security Administration
- ☐ →Veterans Affairs* (burial benefits)

Insurance providers:

- ☐ Health, including Medicare
- ☐ Accident / Life*
- ☐ Home / Renter's
- ☐ Car and other vehicles

Financial {→Money}

- ☐ banks, mortgage lenders, credit card companies*
- ☐ annuity and pension providers*
- ☐ stockbrokers and financial managers*
- ☐ identity protection services*
- ☐ Landlord, Homeowners' Association, Co-op Board*

Communications:

- ☐ Post Office (to whom should mail be forwarded?)
- ☐ Magazine, newspaper, and e-subscriptions
- ☐ Internet and Wireless Server(s)
- ☐ Telephone / →Cell phone services, including Skype
- ☐ Cable TV / Broadband companies
- ☐ Community, advocacy, and religious associations

Domestic

- ☐ utility companies
- ☐ cleaning / gardening services
- ☐ waste disposal

CONFUSION

Yesterday you had come to the bedside with important matters to discuss, questions to ask, and the ill or Departing had been a little subdued but charming, responsive, articulate. Today, she cannot seem to finish a thought or a sentence; he starts up with a heartening enthusiasm, only to peter out moments later.

Problems with →speech are not necessarily evidence of mental confusion. What you interpret as a muddled mind may be muddied neurological pathways to and from the speech centers of the brain, and he may be fully capable of handling complex ideas. Or she may be coping with biomechanical problems of the throat, larynx, and lungs that make speech difficult.

Confusion of mind and stumbling of speech arise from many causes: →pain, painkillers, dehydration, →delirium, long immobility, →depression, general weakness. It's usually more than one cause. Even so, there can be surprising periods of lucidity close to the end. And, despite dehydration, drugs, or a slowed metabolism, some remain lucid throughout.

As hard as it may be to accept an approaching end, it may be harder to accept confusion, for it does not square with the ideal in which the Departing addresses each person at the bedside, in turn, with halting breath but perfect wisdom. {→Last Words}

Those caring for a person with Alzheimer's will be more used to the confusion as it deepens near the end. Those who have been caring for a person with Parkinson's or ALS will be more accustomed to a silence that deepens. Where a disease is not the primary source of the confusion, you may blame yourself for not having come sooner, before the confusion set in, or you may further delay a visit, now that it's no longer certain you will be recognized. Do not blame yourself; do not further delay.

→Crowds and →noise around the bedside aggravate confusion. So do high-intensity conversations. Hint: some sources of confusion are environmental and under your control.

If you are a speedtalker or a mumbler, you will need to remind yourself to speak slowly and strongly. Do not shout or speak in low lugubrious whispers; make an effort to be clear and audible.

The ill and Departing usually realize their difficulty in finding words, and it may upset them to be cued or to have their sentences filled in for them. Frustrated, they may become taciturn, defensive, or scurrilous. At this point it's best to ask yes-and-no questions. You yourself can still talk at length, so long as they like the tenor of your voice, its soundflow.

CONSCIOUSNESS

Of the impending departure? In most cases, the Departing know sooner than you do that they are on the verge of departure; some have a private timetable. {→Anniversaries}

Of those at the bedside? When long-lost friends or grand-nephews suddenly appear at the bedside, the Departing realize that they are expected to pass soon, and that their lives are being recapitulated, calibrated. Or when strangers appear with odd questions about insurance or redemption. Are they aware of you, faithful you, at the bedside day after day? Your faithfulness, yes.

Of goings-on? Less and less. The Departing →hear what is going on and do not expect a constant hush. A hush too prolonged can seem as eerie to them as to us, like a windless silence on a still prairie. Things should be going on. That's life.

Of light, heat, sound, touch? Yes, but with a declining interest in the external sources of their impressions. The work of the Departing may be lost on you; your touch is not lost on them. {→Breastbone}

Of no longer being able to respond? There is sometimes a point several days before departure when the Departing try to respond and realize that they cannot be heard or understood. Their →eyes may register a moment of fright, then settle into another way of looking.

Of being alive? Consider those first few moments of waking from a deep →sleep and a long dream. In what way, exactly, are you alive, and how do you know? What are you sure of? What do you need to be assured of? During Long Days these questions make their way to the surface.

On occasion the serious ill and the Departing may wake after a day or more of near-coma, surprised at being still alive. You will see the surprise in their eyes and may be tempted to say something like, "Well, you're still here," or "Welcome back," which is rather a reassurance for yourself. Instead, wait a bit to see whether they return to sleep; if they do remain awake, say "I'm here" or "We're here," a reassurance of your presence for them, in case they should want something. Do not chatter or try to fill them in on what they have been missing. They are not here for you; you are here for them.

In this regard: I had thought that this would be the chapter in which to address large philosophical questions about the edges between life and death. Guess not.

COUNTDOWNS

9, 8, 7, 6 . . .There is something at once ritualistic and childlike to countdowns, whether to a lift-off or a detonation, the end of a year or the start of a new millennium. Counting down is something that people do together, in sync, to certify and commemorate a moment that is half in and half out of time.

The countdown toward departure is not simply the opposite of a countdown for the launch of a space shuttle, where each system in sequence must be "go"; it is more like the countdown for a game of hide-and-seek: Ready or not, here I come.

Although critical systems in the body may be shutting off in a predictable sequence, each departure has its own rhythm. Hospice workers are familiar with a common if curiously irregular cycling between liveliness and lethargy during the Last Weeks, even the Last Days. That is, the Departing one day may seem to be on the verge of coma, two days later highly responsive, energetic, ravenous. Do not mistake these momentary revivals for a marvelous remission or reprieve. Any countdown toward death is, until the last few hours, nonlinear, something like how a young child counts down: 9, 8, 7, 5, 3, 8, 4, 6, 3, 2, 12, 10, 9, 1 . . . . Ready or not, here I come.

You may suspect that the Departing is pretending for your sake to be far healthier than the prognosis, or grandstanding for the folks from out of town. You may think to yourself (though you would never say so) that it was a waste of time to rush to the bedside just now, and how much more difficult it will be to return in several weeks when the departure is for real. Or you may think that death is not such a remorseless thing if the Departing can play around with it, refit it to a personal calendar {→Anniversaries}.

When the Departing does abide by a countdown, sticking to a tacit schedule, you may suspect that he is trying to the last to be a dutiful parent, or that once again she is the dutiful child. That sense of the obligatory even-unto-death may seem eerie, a consistency beyond reason. . . .What numbers do to us.

Those who choose →not to know the timeline of departure are ordinarily in the company of some who do know but do not say, or have guessed without telling, or have begun a countdown outside the room, which is why so many have shown up from out of state. Soon enough, the Departing who did not want to know may guess exactly where they stand in this numbers-running racket.

Ready or not, here I go.

CRAMPING (musculo-skeletal)

Quinine is more likely to produce blood clots than to relieve muscle cramps. And that's all she wrote. After thousands of years, we know so little about muscle cramps that we cannot explain the exact mechanism or why certain muscles cramp when they do. Nor is there any unfailing remedy.

We do find close, maybe causal associations between cramping and dehydration, whether from heat (and sweating), exercise (and sweating), or the use of diuretics. We find statistical associations between cramping and low blood concentrations of potassium, calcium, magnesium, and sodium, but taking supplements of these does not prevent or mitigate cramps, except perhaps for salt pills. Certain illnesses and procedures are linked specifically to nocturnal leg cramps: vascular issues, lumbar canal stenosis, cirrhosis, →dialysis. Finally, there are confirmed associations with the daily use of naproxen (Alleve), statins (to lower cholesterol), osteoporosis-selective estrogen receptor modulators (for post-menopausal women) and long-acting adrenergic beta agonists (e.g., Serevent, for asthma).

So, for the elderly, the post-menopausal, and athletes who are most prone to recurrent cramping, it's reasonable to keep hydrated, to take salt pills during intense exercise, and possibly to eat a banana for its potassium. Vitamin B12 might also help, but this is unclear, as is the usefulness of eliminating statins or LABAs. We have no solid evidence for the prophylactic value of various stretching or flexibility exercises.

And once cramping has begun, neither water nor salt nor potassium assures relief. Some relief may come from muscle relaxants, an astute massage, hopping on the affected leg, or from heating pads or Vick's VapoRub, or pickle juice, or who knows what else. Whatever works for you. Except quinine.

For *you*. Aside from the spasms of intestinal cramps that are familiar in pregnancy, constipation, appendicitis, gallbladder disease, abdominal cancer, food poisoning, and drug reactions, the Departing or the seriously ill are less likely to be plagued by cramps than you, at the bedside. *You*, who cramp up after →sitting too long in one position and forgetting to drink.

It's thigh, calf, ankle, or toe cramps I'm talking about. One in three adults gets them, especially at night or after long bouts of sitting.

Get up. Walk or skip to a water fountain. Do the hokey-pokey. Whatever works.

CROWDS

Three is a crowd. When it comes to the Last Days, three or four people around the bed can seem like a mob. Imagine yourself weak and half-asleep on morphine, able to hear as usual but unable to focus. What you want is tenderness, peace, quiet, and clarity, not competing voices, faces, motions. So to with the seriously ill and the Departing.

In cases more common during the →Last Months than the Last Days, the Departing may welcome the idea of a party with decorations, cake, and ice cream, and may enjoy hosting such a festive occasion during which friends meet favorite relatives, in less mournful circumstances than a funeral or memorial service.

During the Last Days, the situation is different. Multiple voices, faces, actions and →odors are disconcerting, disorienting. The Departing must summon enormous effort and energy to respond to more than one person at the bedside.

At all costs resist the franticness of crowds. {→Gatekeeping} This means, in practice, that young children should enter the room singly, not in pairs or troupes. That goes for all who prefer to travel in crowds, and for bickering couples.

People who mumble or speak loudly (due to developmental or hearing problems, for example) should be accompanied by someone who can act as a translator or modulator, to clarify or soften the tones. Boisterous people, or those with booming or whining voices, should be cautioned beforehand to speak quietly, lest they seem (as they do elsewhere) a crowd unto themselves.

And that's the point. Crowding is as much a psychological and proprioceptive quality as it is a matter of numbers. Beyond our five senses lies a sixth, proprioception: the bodily sense of the immediately surrounding space and how that is occupied or impinged upon. One person, loud, bumbling, or weeping hysterically, can seem like a crowd; four who work in concert, quietly and efficiently, can seem like one.

During the Last Hours in particular, the Departing require a space to themselves. Our →Last Breaths are all our own, and inevitably must be so. In this sense we all die, and should be allowed to die, alone.

DAUGHTERS AND SONS

Oldest of three sons, I sat at the bedside of my father and my mother. As a lover, I sat at the bedside of a woman who had three daughters. Does the bedside change the relationship between a parent and a child? Among the children? Novelists and playwrights feast upon sibling rivalries at the bedside, revelations made by a father to a son, by a mother to a daughter. Or silences never broken.

And what if it is a son or daughter who is Departing? There are war stories and ghost stories about the deaths of sons and daughters, who are always children to their parents.

And if you are the only child and you are sitting at the bedside, what then? Or the only child, departing? So many tales.

This page is no place for long tales. It is a page, really, for cross-references.

More or less consciously, daughters and sons will be jealous of close friends of their parents who demand too much time at the bedside. Later, they will calibrate their lives by the ages at which their parents died. {→Anniversaries}

They will dance a careful dance with the surviving parent as to the prerogatives of →caregiving, caretaking. These days, however, as people live longer but gradually more frail or limited lives, neither of your parents may be capable of taking care of the other, and you may have to be at two bedsides, one for a departure, the other for long-term "rest." →Mutual incapacities are increasingly common.

Although every child may talk about getting down a parent's life history while there's time, each family usually has one member who walks the talk and records the →History.

Parents may be protective of children, or children of parents, in ways that lead to some knowing more than others about an impending departure, and there will always be things that children choose not to tell a dying parent, following family rules about what is shared and what is kept private.

It's not likely that all daughters or sons will be at the bedside during the →Last Hours, but when some are and some are not, or when an only child is not there, questions about readiness will arise--not just the →readiness of the Departing to depart but the readiness of the child(ren) for the departure of the parent.

Who is letting go of whom?

DEATH AND SURVIVOR BENEFITS

Death Benefit for those already receiving Social Security, from the Social Security website, www.ssa.gov/pubs/deathbenefits.htm

"A one-time payment of $255 is payable to the surviving spouse if he or she was living with the beneficiary at the time of death, OR if living apart, was eligible for Social Security benefits on the beneficiary's earnings record for the month of death." If there is no surviving spouse, payment can be made to a dependent child under the age of 19, or to a dependent parent. This lump-sum payment will come only after notifying Social Security of the death (call 800-772-1213).

Survivors Benefits: www.ssa.gov/pubs/10084.html/10084.pdf: So long as the Departing has not been receiving Social Security (or SSI/Disability) payments and has been part of the workforce for 1.5 years out of the last 3 years, the widow/er and dependent children are eligible for survivors insurance. The benefit amount will depend on age at death, years worked by the deceased, and earnings. A widow/er can receive benefits at any age if taking care of dependent or disabled children of the deceased. "Unmarried children under age 18 (or up to age 19 if attending elementary or secondary school full time) also can receive benefits," as can children who were disabled before age 22 and remain disabled. Those parents who had been receiving at least half their support from the deceased can also receive benefits if age 62+. An ex-wife or ex-husband who is 60 or older can get survivor benefits if the marriage lasted at least 10 years, OR if s/he is currently caring for children of the deceased.

To apply, visit a Social Security office promptly: survivors benefits are sometimes paid starting from the date of application, not the date of death. You must furnish:
--Proof of death, from a funeral home or death certificate;
--Your Social Security number;
--The deceased's Social Security number;
--Your birth certificate;
--Your marriage certificate if a widow/er; divorce papers, if divorced widow/er;
--Dependent children's Social Security numbers, if available;
--Dependent children's birth certificates;
--Deceased's W-2s or self-employed tax return for the most recent year;
--Name of your bank and your account number (for direct deposit).

DEATH AND SURVIVOR BENEFITS, continued

If you are receiving benefits based on your spouse's work, Social Security will change your payments to survivors benefits. If you are getting benefits based on your own work, Social Security will check to see if you can get more money as a widow/er. If you can, you will receive the higher benefit, not both.

A widow/er, at full retirement age or older, receives 100% of the worker's basic benefit amount; over 59 but under full retirement age, 71%-99%; any adult caring for a child under 16, 75%; a child, 75%. Total monthly benefits will be less if you are working while under full retirement age. You do not qualify for widow/er's benefits if you remarry before the age of 60. . . . . Got it?

→See also these related chapters:
Death Certificates
Funeral Arrangements
Obituaries and Obsequies
Paperwork
Veterans
Wives, Husbands, and Lovers

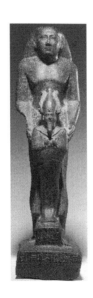

DEATH CERTIFICATES

On signing up for a burial or cremation service, or when the representatives of the service come to pick up the body, you will be asked how many death certificates you want. The Service arranges not only for the preparation and signing of the death certificate but for certified copies to be made. The original of the death certificate is ordinarily included as part of the service. Each copy will cost $10+ and will take a week or more to arrive. The service must wait for a doctor's signature {→Signing Off} and then for processing by the county clerk.

How many certificates will you need? At least six; a dozen if the estate is complex. You may need to supply a separate death certificate in each of the following cases:
--to obtain →Veterans Administration burial benefits;
--to obtain →Death and Survivor Benefits;
--to make a claim on a life insurance policy;
--to transfer shares of stock, bonds, mutual funds (each may require a separate original certificate);
--to amend a revocable trust;
--to rearrange bank accounts (banks need to see an original certificate in order to make their own copy of it).

You may also need to supply (or show) a separate death certificate in these instances:
--to change home/householders insurance;
--to obtain medical records.

It is easier and faster to ask for a sufficient number of copies of death certificates from the burial/cremation service than to try to get them later. Each county has its distinctive process for obtaining copies of death certificates, and new procedures to prevent identity theft have made the issuance of copies more time-consuming.

In most states, only the following are authorized to receive a certified copy of a death certificate: a parent or legal guardian; a child, grandparent, grandchild, sibling, spouse, or legally established domestic partner; an attorney representing the estate; a funeral or mortuary director. Others can request what is called an Informational Copy, which is not a legal document but useful in historical and genealogical research. In any case there will be a fee.

For certified copies of death certificates ordered by snail mail, you will need to obtain a form (often downloadable), sign it in the presence of a notary, mail it along with the notary's certification, and wait several weeks. This entails two separate fees (notarial, county) as well as postage and a delay.

DEATHS, BAD & GOOD, EASY & HARD

No such things.

During the →Last Days, at least, there are no such things. Bad & Good, Easy & Hard, these are judgments *post hoc*. Terms for eulogies.

During the Last Days, there are good hours and bad hours, easy hours and hard hours, for both the Departing and those at the bedside.

Do not hold the Departing, or others at the bedside, to the ideal of a good and easy death. Best practices in end-of-life care, which look toward a good and easy death, are often unavailing, despite the sincerest efforts. The more you take to heart the ideal of a good and easy death, the more you are likely to be disappointed.

Nor is an easy death necessarily a good death. Is a →sudden death a bad death or a good death? Is dying peacefully in one's sleep a good death if one dies alone or unreconciled? Of hunger and dire poverty? A week away from completing a final chapter?

The best and easiest death: dying swiftly and painlessly in the split-second after having done everything one wanted to do. How rare must be such departures. And that best and easiest death does not take into account the enjoyment of one's accomplishments, the love of one's children, friends, students, disciples, carriers-on.

We might agree on the criteria of a hard death: great →pain, →anxiety, dark hallucinations, loss of control of one's bodily functions, cruel abandonment, torture. Hard deaths are more common than any of us would like to imagine, less common than the most pessimistic among us fear.

Is a hard death necessarily a bad death? Each religious tradition and each warring community has martyrs for its cause whose hard deaths are celebrated as good deaths.

None of this helps much at the bedside. At the bedside one helps the Departing toward a departure that should be free from regret. Free from if-only's: *If only he could stick around for another month to finish the sculpture . . . If only we could give her something right now to make her articulate, so we could understand what she is trying to tell us. . . .* Why surround dying with the aggravation of despair and recriminations of remorse? Enough is going on otherwise.

DELIRIUM

Delirium occurs in such various circumstances that it is not definitive of any illness, but in and of itself delirium can be dangerous, even fatal. It can be at once the cause and result of neurobiological changes, including a metabolic disturbance or shortage of oxygen that injures brain cells.

So whether it's the result of a morphine overdose or a reaction to sedatives, of high fever or heart attack, of urinary tract infections or kidney dysfunction or dehydration, it must be attended to. As Jane Brody of the *New York Times* has written in "Vigilance About the Dangers of Delirium," (10/1/2012), "At least one in five hospital patients over sixty-five experiences delirium related complications, some of which--like worsened dementia--may never completely resolve."

Since rates and severity of delirium increase where people already at risk are physically and geographically disoriented, as in recovery from surgery or in →intensive care units, those at the bedside should make every effort, ASAP, to reorient a patient to place, time, familiar faces and objects. Playing favorite pieces of →music, or going through family photos may also help, as will occupational and physical therapy to improve mobility and decrease isolation.

A good night's →sleep is crucial. This means that if a patient has been going in and out of the hyperactive or depressive states characteristic of some forms of delirium, you will need to push strongly for a private room or for a change of semi-private rooms in those cases where a →roommate is coughing, moaning, screaming, shouting for help, or watching loud tv.

Be sure to get second opinions before allowing staff to administer those sedatives customarily used to calm patients who are agitated, confused, or hallucinatory. Many sedatives, muscle relaxants, and painkillers deepen delirium. The current preferred treatment is to keep a delirious patient awake, aware, engaged, and reassured.

Delirium is one of the few instances in which restraints are still used to protect patients from themselves or from falling out of bed. However, such restraints also have a record of deepening delirium and producing recurrent nightmares. If you can be at the bedside overnight, you may be able to persuade hospital or SNF staff not to strap on the restraints.

Delirium can subside or suddenly disappear. If however it continues, work closely with physicians, nurses, and therapists. Your presence is significant.

DEPRESSION

Losing your appetite? Losing weight? Losing track of mealtimes?

Losing →sleep? Sleeping too much? Unable to sleep at all? Dreamless, or awakened again and again by nightmares?

Losing track of the days? Forgetting what happened an hour ago? Neglecting to return phone calls? To pay your bills?

Perseverating? Ruminating? (That is, caught in a spiral of thoughts--of regret, of recrimination, of despair, of anger and grief--you cannot seem to escape?)

Unable to find the humor in much of anything? Uninterested in news, gossip, rumor, secrets confided or revealed?

Anxious to the point of panic? Always about to weep?

Speaking less than usual? Avoiding conversation?

Distracted, so much that you can't focus on a movie or a book or a favorite show or on what someone is telling you just now?

If you nodded yes to several of the above, you are depressed. You need help. Now. And not from a how-to book or article, not from over-the-counter drugs or a friend's →medicine cabinet. You need to talk to someone. Today.

Isolation is the issue. The more depressed you are, the more you isolate yourself. You flee. Into yourself. Not a good idea. Where isolation is the issue, you are no remedy for yourself.

You say to yourself: of course I'm depressed. The person I love most in the world is in terrible jeopardy, or dying. I am at the bedside to be of help, but it's only human to feel →sad when you see a loved one in such pain or slipping away. It'll take time, but I'll be OK. Don't worry about me.

Postures and rhetorics of martyrdom are a form of →blackmail at the bedside. Face it, you can be of no help at the bedside when you are depressed. A paradox, to be sure: you arrive to be company and comfort, to reduce the isolation of someone you love, and you end up in a personal isolation ward. This is a case of →mutual peril, and a common casualty of →caregiving.

Depression is at root (again, paradoxically) a social disease. Feeling for each other, we are so overwhelmed by the tragedy or complexity of situations out of our hands that we turn in upon ourselves. The cure is equally social: returning to the world, to the voice and warmth of others.

DETAILS

Always perplexing during the Last Days is how and why the Departing are still preoccupied with minutiae: a loose thread, a button misbuttoned, the angle of a lampshade, the position of eyeglasses on a bed table. For goodness sake, these are the Last Days, and the Departing surely have more important things to attend to than whether you put one of those small packets of nutrients into the vase of cut flowers to keep them in bloom a while longer. A bad example, those flowers; the analogy is too apparent.

That's the point. During the Last Days, the Departing find in their collapsed environs a host of small things that are microcosms of larger issues. Their immediate world may be smaller and enclosed; their minds, their memories may remain expansive. So all of life is now in the little things. {→Doodads}

Not everything, of course, is charged with symbolism. A mosquito is a mosquito, annoying as at any other bedtime.

Further, the Departing may have been obsessive while alive-- nail-biters, bean counters, number crunchers. You would like to think that during the Last Days they would shake off that obsessiveness, that compulsiveness. Hah.

Are they grabbing for what lies within reach, not so much to hold on for dear life as to be reassured that they, and their lives, are still material: bone unto bone china, ring finger unto ring?

Do you try to get the Departing back on track for a meaningful departure, or do you find in each gesture or word of the Departing a mortal significance? What else justifies, really, your coming to the bedside and staying there? If not a guide, if not an interpreter, what are you? And what have they, the Departing, been doing all the while, when so much hangs in the balance? Isn't this bedside gambit supposed to be a collective effort toward insight or love? What does a fork with a bent tine have to do with insight or love?

Exasperated as you may become with such finickiness, there is nothing for it. Who are you to tell the Departing what dying is supposed to be about? Everyone else has at least one foot in the humdrum, even during the Last Days; why not also the Departing?

Could be, too, that there is an amazing secret insight behind his infinite concern with the arrangement of a straw, or a vital life-clue in her continual rearranging of the bedclothes. Or not. {Or →Floccillation}

DIALYSIS

Strictly speaking, the cleansing of toxins from the →blood safely extends life, and dialysis patients are not bedridden, so dialysis should not be a headliner in this book, but the annual mortality for Americans on dialysis is one in five, and those who start dialysis after age sixty can expect to live on average another 4.5 years. The severe mortality is due in part to illnesses consociated with renal failure, such as diabetes, congestive heart failure, and peripheral vascular disease.

Whether done daily by oneself at home or thrice weekly by technicians at a center, dialysis is a lifelong commitment. Only 4% who begin dialysis ever go off it: those whose healthy kidneys were briefly compromised by systemic infection or injury, and those who receive a kidney transplant. In the US, about 400,000 people are on dialysis; worldwide, 2,000,000.

Dialysis engages caregivers as helpmeets with →tubing and →needles at home or as drivers to local centers, but especially as cooks, since it entails a diet restricting salt, potassium (K), and phosphorus (P), which quickly build up in the blood of those with kidney failure and may cause fatigue, breathing problems, joint pain, irregular heartbeats, muscle spasm or paralysis. Renal diets are fierce balancing acts, since they require substantial protein, most forms of which are stuffed with K. Vegetarians must struggle all the more, since nuts, seeds, soy, and whole grains are high in both K and P. Those doing daily home dialysis will have an easier time: more frequent dialysis filters out more of the salt, K, and P. All can benefit from liquid protein supplements for renal diets (Nepro, Renalcal, Suplena, Novasource). Most on dialysis will also take prescribed phosphate blockers (or "binders") with each meal to prevent the absorption of P.

Dialysis patients are not bedridden, so you won't be at a person's bedside just because s/he is on dialysis. Indeed, cruise ships now offer "dialysis cruises."

Nonetheless, dialysis is a serious matter. Someone who misses a week, just three sessions, of dialysis is likely to be near-death, even when attending to diet and keeping well hydrated. That's how quickly toxins build up in the blood of those with end-stage (=stages IV and V) kidney disease. Other infections, diseases, and injuries can also and immediately undermine the effectiveness of dialysis.

More? National Kidney Foundation (www.kidney.org / 800 622 9010); www.billpeckham.com/from_the_sharp_end_of_the/

DIAPERS {also →Shit Happens}

Few now are the seriously ill and Departing lucky enough to spend their time abed without diapers and their peripherals: mattress protectors, waterproof sheeting or underpads (e.g., Chux); →gloves and wipes at the bedside, and talcum powder, lotion for the perineum, baby oil, a dedicated waste receptacle.

Near the end, incontinence is more or less to be expected, but depending on prior surgeries, stroke, or paralysis, it may have begun well before. Bedside regulars soon take it in stride.

For newcomers, seeing a parent or sibling in diapers is one of the greater shocks of the Last Days. Diapers can be equally shocking, and humiliating, for those among the Departing who had managed their own toileting until, say, a week ago. Hospice workers find that it is common for people who have not been out of bed for days to try silently and valiantly to get themselves down off a mattress so that they can walk to a bathroom. Some, less precipitate, ask for strong arms to assist, and may consent to using the more public, bedside commode. In either case, once down out of bed they invariably collapse, even with help, and end up on the floor, usually unhurt but sobbing in despair. Which is why hospice nurses advise those at the bedside not to let the Departing inveigle them into such a trek. But how can you not want to help a person whose final assertion of physical independence is a trip to the toilet?

Adult diapers are icons of infantilization and a return to dependency. When someone is in acute crisis or intermittently conscious, diapers won't register as deeply as in periods of recuperation, when the changing of diapers becomes an issue more emotional than physical. Those abed and at the bedside may then both prefer the practiced assistance of strangers, hired hands {→Caregivers--Hiring}.

If you end up as the one ordering incontinence supplies, you may need schooling in diapers, whose variety can befuddle:
--washable cloth?... or plasticized disposables, which in the long run are ecologically problematic but less hassle?
--pull-up/step-in?. . . or open-side/wrap-around, which are easier to change but not much good if a person is up and about
--super absorbent, highly absorbent, or normal?
--purchases at a discount store? . . . or automatic delivery of cases to your doorstep, cheaper but likely to result in a bulky surplus exactly when you don't want to think about such things.

As if you had ever wanted to think about the nexus between diapers and death.

DIMINISHING

Traditional images of the sickbed show the patient becoming thinner and smaller. With many diseases, however, people swell up, become visibly larger, violating the aesthetics of the Last Days. The fatness of the dying seems to defeat the purpose of your presence. You came to be at the bedside of someone disappearing.

Cirrhosis of the liver, portal vein thrombosis, hepatitis, liver cancer, pancreatic cancer, ovarian cancer, congestive heart failure, and tuberculosis are often accompanied by ascites. Once called abdominal dropsy,→ascites is a swelling due to an accumulation of fluid in the peritoneal cavity between the abdominal organs and abdominal lining.

Peripheral edema is also likely for those who have been bedridden for a week or more, or with lymphatic problems. Mechanical sleeves or cuffs are now available that automatically apply intermittent pressure to the limbs in order to reduce the probability of swelling and consequent skin irritation and pain.

None of this is easy to deal with. You want the departing to be recognizable during the Last Days {→Accidentals; Identity}. You say to yourself, the body is not the person; but it is hard to separate the cognizable from the recognizable, the spirit from the flesh, when there is so much more flesh apparent. It would be more compatible with the etiquette of dying if the body in the bed were shrinking, as if the inner light of the person could shine without being obscured by its mortal cloak. Instead, you are distracted by the swelling. How foolish, how petty of you to be thinking these thoughts when there is so little time left for more vital matters.

Some come to the bedside as morticians to a corpse, taking it as their job to make the departing presentable for departure. They struggle the most against the ascites, the edema, the swelling. They comb the hair and lay out the most attractive outfits, preparing the frame, as it were, for a final studio portrait. They believe that their attentions are as welcome and necessary as their intentions are good. Theirs is a way of coping that does not require too much thought, a kind of painting-by-number. In the mid-nineteenth century, people asked photographers to take pictures of them lying next to the departed, or with a dead child, beautifully dressed, in their arms.

Death need not diminish us.

DIRECTIVES, ADVANCE, AND OTHERWISE

Apart from suicide, death used to be out of our hands and, often, out of the hands of →physicians, who were better at mitigation than cure. As drugs became more predictably effective and complex surgeries safer, physicians began to believe that they had more power over death, and people began to put more trust in that power once they commonly began to live to an age where death results from degenerative diseases or chronic conditions. Had my father been born in 1900 rather than 1920, he would have died of a stroke at the age of fifty-nine, colon cancer at sixty-eight, a viral infection of the spine at seventy-four. He lived to be eighty-seven.

So now we make our wishes for our departure known ahead of time not only to family and friends but to doctors and hospitals, lest our deaths be taken out of our hands and shaped by the newest drugs and technologies. Ironic, isn't it? We compose directives often opposing the use of "extraordinary measures" to prolong our lives because we have come to appreciate (and fear?) the extraordinary progress that has been made in prolonging our lives during medical →emergency.

When you fill out an Advance Health Care Directive, for which forms are available in hospitals, on the web, and in state offices, you dictate: (1) What, if any, measures should be taken to prolong your life when terminally ill, permanently unconscious, or otherwise in need of life-sustaining treatment; (2) Who will speak for you if you are unable to make medical decisions for yourself. (You can and should designate a series of people to speak for you, should the first person on the list be unavailable. You cannot designate your own physician.)

Physicians now also work with a POLST form, which both doctor and patient sign after mutual discussion, especially with regard to treatment goals and limits in progressive illness. These Physician Orders for Life-Sustaining Treatment do much the same as Advance Health Care Directives but explicitly engage a patient's primary doctor and can often be counted on to be more exactly honored.

A Living Will is a less complete form of an advance directive; like the Natural Death Act Declaration of years past, it deals only with terminal illness or coma. It does not address other situations, and it does not designate anyone to speak for you.

DIRECTIVES, ADVANCE, AND OTHERWISE, continued

A Durable Power of Attorney for Health Care is an advance directive that explicitly identifies the person(s) who will speak for you should you become incapacitated or unconscious. It does not necessarily or extensively detail your wishes with regard to extraordinary measures.

All four directives are legal in most states without needing to be officially filed, so long as you are of age (18). A few states require them to be notarized. In any case, you must sign and date them, your signature witnessed by two others, neither of whom can be a person designated to speak for you.

You may change or cancel your directives at any time, even in the hospital, so long as you are of sound mind. Any oral changes should be made in the presence of two people, perhaps an attending physician and a family member, to avoid subsequent controversy.

Save copies of any/all of these documents in a fireproof box. Also distribute copies of these documents to all who may be closely involved in your care--physicians, visiting nurses, friends, kin, longtime caregivers.

Emergency rooms and hospitals now ask for copies of Advance Directives as a matter of course for those with life-threatening illnesses, or undergoing surgery or blood transfusion, or when considered candidates for hospice. And they do not save these directives. Each time you return to the same ER or hospital, they will ask you yet again for a copy of the directive.

See also
→Acuteness
→DNR (Do Not Resuscitate)
→Power of Attorney
→Urgency

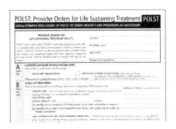

DNR (Do Not Resuscitate)

Do Not Resuscitate means just what it says: under no circumstances should doctors, paramedics, or anyone else try to revive a person who is failing. No extraordinary measures should be taken to keep the person alive--no CPR, no IVs.

During the Last Days in general, and by contractual rule with →hospices, no one should call 911 on behalf of the Departing. If there is severe breakthrough pain or profuse bleeding, call hospice directly, or a physician, or a duty nurse.

Hospices require that the Departing have DNR orders posted around the house--on the refrigerator, bedstead, even the front door. Such an order can also be put into a medical chart in hospitals and posted above a bed in →skilled nursing facilities.

Paramedics responding to a 911 call are not obliged to look for or ask about a DNR order. They will proceed with CPR even when it has no chance of success (as in cases of septic shock, metastasized cancer, renal failure, AIDS). So if a DNR is in place but by mistake they have been called to the bedside, they must immediately be shown the DNR order.

Agreeing to a DNR is usually done by the Departing in talks with physicians, family, lovers. Often the Departing initiates the process, exhausted by a series of painful procedures, failed trials, or long stays in hospital. It can be more harrowing when kin or lifelong friends initiate the process, since no one can avoid second doubts while urging a loved one toward a shorter life. Further, those who have endured a severe chronic illness for years have a different take on →"quality of life" than those who shudder at the prospect. In any case, a physician must sign the DNR {→Directives}.

On legal and ethical issues surrounding coma, persistent vegetative state, and brain death, see→Further Reading.

Deciding upon a DNR is a necessary but never a sufficient factor in determining the start of the →Last Days, since the Departing may be fragile but remain on an even keel for weeks or months after the issuance.

DNR orders may be hardest on those in denial, who refuse to acknowledge that the death of a loved one is so near as to require such a heartless command: "Do Not Resuscitate." {→Stages}

Do Not Resuscitate never means Do Not Reconsider. DNR orders can be rescinded. Any time, any place, for any reason. I take that back: no reason need be given.

DOODADS

Things take on an enormous weight at the bedside, and I am not pontificating about the momentousness of your presence. I mean, literally, *things*: appliances, accessories, devices, gadgets, gimcracks, doodads.

An alphabetical list of some of these things may make the point: alphabet boards, bath chairs, blood glucose monitors, canes, commodes, CPAP machines, drinking straws, exercise spirometers, foot rests, gait belts, Hoyer lifts, intermittent leg compression devices (ICDs), jars of cotton swabs, kleenex, low-pressure air mattresses, mechanical grabbers, nightlights, overbed tables, pressure-relieving heel-protecting boots, quiet floor fans, remote controls, slide boards, stretch bands with variable resistance levels, toilet safety frames, underwear bags, vaseline, wheelchairs, workstations for the lap(top).

Chances are that you will come back from the hospital with many of these in tow and strict instructions to get/install others. If Medicare is involved, and a hospital →case manager, much of the haul (known as Durable Medical Equipment) will be free. If not, you will need to balance expense against sanitary priorities when purchasing (on Craig's List or elsewhere) used *things*.

There is much to be said individually for each doodad, but altogether they may weigh down a room and make your hours at the bedside seem onerous. (Unless you are an engineer or gadgeteer, in which case they furnish endless amusement.) Learning how each one works, studying which type is most affordable, this in itself is time-consuming. But the real risk is that a mob of doodads can get in the way of making eye contact at the bedside, of holding a hand, or listening closely. So much to do, so many *things* to remember. . . .

I could devote an entire manual to the ins-and-outs of these *things*. Someday maybe I will. Here I want to note that a seriously ill person may like the feeling of command that comes from a mastery of doodads. Nearer to departure, however, *things* do get in the way and should be removed wherever possible. Exercise bands will be among the first to go; the sippy cup last. And you may find yourself using the grabber until the very end, to retrieve other *things* that have fallen into awkward corners.

That is the nature of *things*: to fall into awkward corners. Never let things put you in an awkward corner with the Departing or with others at the bedside. *Things* are not worth the trouble (which is why I have been calling them "doodads").

EMERGENCIES

OK, let's get this sorted out. Once the →Last Days have been reached, all crises are past. There can be no emergencies. Death itself, under these conditions, is not a crisis.

Yet those who now come to the bedside may arrive outfitted for emergency. They have changed travel plans, taken time off from work, asked in-laws to tend to children or pets. They have an idea that they can be effective. Even when the Departing is with a →hospice and has posted →DNR forms in every room, they believe that they will have jobs to do upon arrival, things that must be managed without delay.

Florence Nightingale, in her no-nonsense *Notes on Nursing*, was a partisan of efficiency, but she disliked hurry and bustle because she found that her patients were more upset by an atmosphere of strain than by the fact of illness, however grim, and necessary procedures, however painful.

Those who come to the bedside in the ready-for-anything mode are often ready for everything but the departure. When there is quiet, they tend to look for something, *anything*, to do. When there is something to do, they do it too fast, or without consultation. A while back, when there were major decisions to be made during the Long Days, you could have used these visitors as one uses an emergency preparedness unit. Now, their zeal feels like posturing, as if they can tolerate the Last Days only so long as they become action figures, drawing up →checklists, making "arrangements."

True, some arrangements may need to be made, but most have probably been set in motion already, and the rest must wait until the Days After. And true, there are always little errands, which they will gratefully run. They came to the bedside to be *busy*. Do they mean to give the Departing the bum's rush toward death? No, though that's how it may appear as they check schedules, smart phones, tablets. Do they mean to treat the Departing like a passenger in a first-class lounge? No, although by their demeanor that's how it may appear. (Do you want anything at all before boarding? *Anything* at all?)

During the Last Days no one, and everyone, is out of time. These are liminal days, outside the normal run of time, when one can →sit with another in silence and not worry about the minutes. And if you are going to sit by the bedside, wrote Nightingale, do not fidget.

ENTERTAINMENT

Comedies seem to be the preferred genre for those on the mend. But →Laughter can be therapeutic throughout a long decline, and even during the Last Days a joke may not be amiss. The Departing herself may be quick with black humor.

Be advised, however, that until the very end those abed may wish to keep hold of issues more momentous than mistaken identities, witticism, and slapstick. He may want to be a full, knowledgeable participant in discussions of the daily news; she will be impatient with chitchat about the weather or coupons.

During the Last Days, the Departing is neither invested in, nor much amused by, the human comedy. She generally does not want to watch melodramas or reality shows. She tends to prefer quietness, or short conversation, or particular kinds of →music (not necessarily soulful, Contemplative or Meditative--learn her preferences). If you play an instrument, this may be welcome; ask.

If your efforts to entertain the Departing are ignored or dismissed, do not feel bad.

Or, feel bad. Feel bad if you impose some entertainment upon the Departing because you are bored, anxious, unable to express your own concerns, or trying to drown out the cries of pain or the hard breathing of death.

During the Last Days time passes differently for the Departing than for you, and entertainment for the sake of "passing the time" is morbidly redundant. If you want to watch a DVD at the bedside, do not pretend it is for the sake of the Departing. The Departing already have their programs.

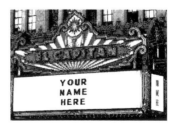

ETD (Estimated Time of Departure)

Parlor game: If you had 24 hours to live, what would you do? A fantasy. With months to live, the seriously ill have many workable wishes. During the Last Days, few.

Lesson One: Before it's too late, act to help the Departing visit places of their dreams, see friends, speak truth to power. It may be awkward, expensive, complicated--all weak reasons to defer what may seem more like an expedition than a trip.

Lesson Two: If not a parlor game, the ETD is a guessing game. Doctors are always asked, "How long does he have? Should I send for the family? Will she be conscious a week from now?" No one likes to answer these questions, although →hospices work only with those certified "terminal" within six months. Home nurses and physicians know that six months is a guess, as is five weeks or three days, and all have stories of delayed departure, stunning remissions, sudden declines {→Cascades}.

Lesson Three: The longer the ETD (nine months, two years), the less reliable.

Lesson Four: The ETD is a lottery with side-effects. The more distant the ETD, the more likely there will be untoward consequences, and a progressively restricted or painful life {→Quality of Life} Clinical studies of experimental drugs or procedures in end-stage diseases are reported in terms of the percentage of subjects who survive for x months afterward. If 50% survive for nine months longer than control subjects who do not get the drugs or procedure, that's often accounted a success, but read the small print: how many dropped out because of bad side effects; how many died before their time?

Or say the ETD puts the Departing squarely within the last month. Then what? Go for a second opinion, to lengthen the ETD? Go for experimental procedures, ditto? Go for broke at the racetrack? Buy eighty lottery tickets? Call the extended family back from vacations or from across the country? Call in the →lawyers? It all depends on what you take an ETD to be: a reluctant prophecy, a gambler's odds, or a judicial verdict. Each is reversible, and each can be awfully wrong.

Lesson Five: we have no lock on time, but it's one of the last things over which we willingly give up our putative control. Take the ETD, then, as a cue to forget the calendar and get on with the necessary conversations. Those are more or less under our control, and never a gamble.

ETHICAL WILLS

What do you say at the bedside?

Do you gossip about friends, neighbors, celebrities? Do you gripe about work? Do you enthuse over vacation travel or good →music? Do you reminisce? Do you debate politics or swap philosophies of life? Do you play word games aloud or labor together over crosswords? Or do you run through Twenty Questions on things medical, hospital, and pharmaceutical?

Whatever pleases the both of you. Both. If one or the other is bored, exasperated, or stubbornly silent, move on or get out of the room. Never cater to each other's obsessions, never foster perseveration (the repetition of an idea or phrase). Do not keep up a conversation if it's making hearts pound, heads throb.

A healthy topic for returning conversations, during Long Days as in the Last Months, is the fashioning of an Ethical Will.

Unlike standard →wills, Ethical Wills concern not material property but moral propriety, not deeds to land or houses but deeds of hospitality and charity, not financial shares and investments but what it means to share and how to invest in friendships, loves, family, community, society.

What a person puts in an Ethical Will is itself fodder for continuing conversation. An Ethical Will is a considered declaration of one's central principles to be shared with friends and family as a legacy of one's values. It need not be a religious document. It need not be elegant or logically self-consistent. It may be a series of aphorisms, or a set of pointed questions, or a parable. It need not be written in indelible ink-- yea, it could be drawings, cartoons, songs.

What it shouldn't be is flippant, borrowed, or plagiarized. It can be playful, but it should also be thoughtful, thought-provoking, and a person's *own*. Your conversation will elicit dilemmas, and you don't have to agree in order to continue on toward completion. In fact, if you both agree on everything, then something is wrong, the Ethical Will is not a person's *own*.

As much as an Ethical Will reasons rather than teases, it also exhorts rather than extorts, supposes rather than imposes. It is something to live up to, and for. It is about the past, the present, and a lively future. It is not about death or dying, and it is not a form of →blackmail.

It will take some time. At the bedside during the Long Days and Last Months, you have time.

EXCUSES AND CARDS

Excuses seem irrelevant, if not inept, during the →Last Days, since excuses oscillate in the cloudy region between either and or, while the Last Days insist on binaries. Either you are at the bedside, or not.

What excuses you from the bedside?
---The critical illness of another, especially a child.
---Physical inability to travel.
---Your own illness, if debilitating, obnoxious, or infectious.
---Your own emotional instability or fragility, due to the recent departure of another or your own recent brush with death.
---Your own psychological problems, if likely to be exacerbated by scenes during the Last Days, or if likely to prove dangerous to the Departing.
---Great distance, and poverty.

If you cannot come, call. Better still, write a good long letter that can be →read in parts and reread in sentences. Best, send your own art, photos, or craftwork along with a letter. Consider these as conversations or meditations.

As for cards, these are tricky. Hope You Are Feeling Better? Get Well Soon? Happy 50th? Belated Greetings? Best Wishes? Oops? My Sincerest. . . .

Candy, if you send it, is not really for the seriously ill or the Departing, but she may like the opportunity for largesse, offering pieces to visitors, and he may decide to make a gift of an unopened box to the nurses' station or to an aide. Dark chocolates, with 60% or more cocoa, may be welcome to sleepy caregivers because they contain 75-150 mg of caffeine per 100 grams, which is as much as in a small cup of espresso (75 mg) or a Starbucks Tall Caffè Americano (150 mg).

Flowers may momentarily cheer up those at the bedside, or not. (Some hospitals now discourage them, and some people at home are allergic.) If a space is small, they will be in the way, or be taken away.

It's best not to use flowers or candy or printed cards or giftshop gifts as outflung elements of an excuse ("sorry I could not be there, could not stay longer, could not find my own words, could not tear myself away from work or family..."). These can easily seem *pro forma*.

The power of forgiveness is neither in the departure nor in the Departing but in the staying on: what is it, after all, that you want excused? Not stopping for death?

EXPOSURE

After weeks of care at hospital, →hospice, or →home, the seriously ill and the Departing have been exposed to so many eyes and touched by so many strangers' hands under so many situations usually private that privacy--and sometimes gender itself--can no longer have the same coordinates. They may shed concerns about modesty but resist all the more fiercely the invasiveness of unwanted visitors {→Gatekeeping}. Or those at the bedside may assert on their behalf a prudery neither personally characteristic nor currently practical. Conversely, those in bed may shock (and eventually bore) those at the bedside who innocently ask "How are you today?" with accounts of hard-won bowel movements, →catheter reinsertions, itches in almost inaccessible places.

Long Days and extended departures entail such exposure that you may wonder whether "death with dignity" is possible. In sheerly physical terms, is dignity a philosopher's mirage? If an inviolate space around one's body is basic to the notion of dignity, then none with extended departures will ever be allowed to die with dignity. If dignity has to do with command of one's immediate direction and destiny, then it behooves those at the bedside to consult with the ill and the Departing on all choices medical, social, economic, and environmental.

Worse than the loss of bodily shame may be the forced abandonment of sensibilities, such that those abed are compelled to lie exposed to colors or →music they abhor, to voices whose timbres are nervewracking, to a stickiness at which they have shuddered since childhood. One of the subtler skills of the bedside is to identify these sorts of →exposure and, where feasible, eliminate them {→Odors, Ugliness}.

As for emotional exposure, this you are likely to share with those abed. Even at home, feelings of vulnerability lead caregivers to ignore ringing phones, avoid newspapers, reroute televisions from the six o'clock news, and generally wall off the bedside from intrusions of public travails. This often occurs prematurely, before the ill or Departing are ready to call it quits on the outside world. Caretakers may go to such extremes as to insulate them not only from news of natural disasters and human violence but from news of the passing of relatives, friends, or even (as happened with my father's father) the passing of his wife in another facility. The moral issues surroundings such extreme protectiveness and extreme feelings of vulnerability are profound and must be talked through. Silence is no reliable guide to the wisdom of silence.

EYES

Looking toward months of recuperation, or in the toils of illness, people tend to neglect eye exams and stick with eyeglasses now too weak or out of whack from ageing, stress, disease. Although the old glasses are useless for watching tv or movies and cause headaches when reading, a trip to an optometrist may be considered too strenuous and trivial given everything else that is going on. Unless beset by eye infections, the ill may also downplay the ophthalmic side-effects of drugs-- itching, blurred vision, sensitivity to →light (caused by tetracycline, tricyclic anti-depressants, and blood pressure regulators) or the growth of cataracts (from high-dose steroids).

But functional blindness to the world beyond arm's length should not be acceptable collateral damage of the Long Days. Make every effort to help the seriously ill get better eyeglasses, or at least large-print books, and seek medical help with eye problems.

During the Last Weeks and Days, the eyes of the Departing may be open but glassy or wandering. Or they may be lightly shut. The eyes can become dry and itchy from lack of tear duct secretions. If you notice the Departing rubbing at any eye, or if you spot a crust forming around an eye, ask for eyedrops to reduce dryness and itching.

You too must be careful of your eyes, which can become infected after →weeping or eye-rubbing, or dried out in critical-care rooms where air is artificially circulated.

Since we tend to read each other by the movement, focus, and color of the eyes, a slow loss of clarity of vision and loss of interest in keeping the eyes open become particularly sad instances of an approaching departure. If however the eyes appear to be tightly closed and the brow furrowed, this is more likely a sign of →pain than of withdrawal, and you need to get the morphine. If the eyes are open but evidently frightened or preoccupied, you are dealing with visions, waking dreams, and →ghosts that commonly appear to the Departing during the Last Days.

At the end, the Departing do not necessarily close their eyes. Their eye sockets may be dark and taut, but in death the eyes can remain slightly open. The eyelids may relax to such an extent that the eyes are fully open and clear. Sometimes (for a few minutes or an hour or so), they may even be radiant.

FALLING

"Fall we all." A common line from early American school primers and alphabet books, rehearsing a Calvinist notion of original sin and harking back to the Book of Genesis.

Fall Risk. A common sign posted behind beds in hospitals and →skilled nursing facilities. Often accompanied by bed rails or alarms (lest a person who is weak, →confused, or →delirious try to get out of bed without help).

Each year, one in three adults age 65+ falls, but less than half of the fallen tell their doctors about it (so we are told by the Centers for Disease Control). Falls can cause hip fractures and brain damage, and may increase the risk of early death. Among the elderly, falls are the leading cause of injury death and the most common cause of hospital admissions for trauma.

Also, "Many people who fall, even if they are not injured, develop a fear of falling. This fear may cause them to limit their activities, which leads to reduced mobility and loss of physical fitness, and in turn increases their actual risk of falling."

One way or another, then, human frailty catches us up into a circle of jeopardy, which must be offset by a circle of caring. Offset in three ways, as follows.

One. Since those who fall may keep their falling secret lest their independence be lost, they need a community that sustains them in such a manner that they feel safe revealing their falls--a circle that does not automatically associate physical falling with failure or a decline into senility.

Two. Since those inclined to fall often simply collapse without injury, they may need to be rescued (returned to vertical or to bed) without medical attention, so they need a community that can respond quickly and adeptly to calls for help without inducing anxiety, raising further alarms, or calling 911.

Three. Since those inclined to fall should take preventive measures, they need a circle of care to convince them to: exercise regularly; use a walker; review all medications for side effects of dizziness; get →eye exams and apt eyeglasses; remove throw rugs from the home; install grab bars in the tub or shower and next to the toilet; and perhaps contract with a company that provides bracelet or necklace call buttons and a communication system at home for getting help after a fall. Outside the home, they need a simple →cell phone with quick-call capabilities to reach the circle of care.

All of this, of course, is intended to avert Long Days.

FATIGUE

Admit it, during the first hours/days of a medical →emergency, you find yourself in a kind of mania compounded of dread, dare, and excitement. Your competence and endurance are being challenged toward the noblest of ends. And you are up to it. Of course you are. You have to be.

But then . . . but then. As the days become weeks, weeks months, months perhaps years of attendance at the bedside, filling water pitchers, mopping up spills, changing soiled sheets, charging →upstairs and down, you tire. As a principal →caregiver, your love and loyalty are not in question but your enthusiasm dwindles, your devotion almost autonomous.

Even if you do not get →depressed, do not lose sleep or appetite (or eat too much and stop exercising); and even if you need not worry about money, work, or business; and even if there are no pressing family matters; and even if the house needs no repairs and your car is a workhorse wonder; and even if all the pets and plants indoors and out are thriving; even so, you are in for it: exhaustion.

Spell that with a lower-case *e*, exhaustion, because it creeps up on you, and either you sleep for three days straight or you become crabby and/or →forgetful and/or careless and/or ill.

This is not because you are constitutionally weak or eating too few anti-oxidants or drinking too much coffee. It's because you are human. True, over-caffeination does not help, but your exhaustion is as much mental, spiritual, aesthetic, and emotional as it is physical or chemical. You need →respite. And you need to realize that if you do not take some time away, you will be doing everyone a disservice, including the person in his Last Months or the Departing in her Last Days.

If you are not a principal caregiver, you may find yourself coming to the bedside less frequently. With the initial mania long gone, all that's left is some inertial momentum, which you may come to resent. Sometimes you may secretly hope (very secretly, because it feels inexcusable) for a little medical excitement, something to get your heart racing as you hasten to the bedside--something important and immediate for you to do. My suggestion: make yourself available as a week-long respite caregiver, and insist that the principal caregiver take the offered respite, all the while assuring everyone that you have no intention of usurping relationships or stealing love. (Yes, such assurances are necessary.)

This handbook is entirely opposed to martyrdom.

FEAR OF DEATH

Philosophers and biologists put us in an unenviable position: we are the only beings who know we are going to die, yet we share with other living beings an instinct for survival that is sometimes overcome by compassion, sometimes by desires for the continuity of family, tribe, ethnos, nation. Does foreknowledge of our mortality make us therefore more fearful or less fearful of death? And the closer we come to our departures, are we hence more resigned or more rebellious?

One way or another, systems of religion and metaphysics attempt to defuse the fear of death, especially for those who have lived a long, good life. Because none of us enjoys a guarantee of long life or any assurance that we have done all we could for others while alive, death can be frightening at any time. And because frailty, immobility, and irreducible →pain can come upon us at any time, death can also be welcome.

During Long Days and at the Last Days, we at the bedside must release the seriously ill and the Departing from any obligations either toward heroism or fairytale optimism, lest we cause further suffering. But we need not suppress our own fears of death or our anger or →sadness at one more life cut short.

The Departing often come to terms with their departure before the rest of us. When we talk about the fear of death during the Last Days, we need to be clear and direct about who is afraid, who is not. {→Apples and Oranges; Frankness.}

This is not a question of solace.

FEET {also →Shoes}

Ethnographers have reached no consensus on the origins or significance of the oiling and rubbing of feet, although this occurs in ritual and in relaxation across the world, in places of diverse temperature and temperament. There is no reason to abandon the practice during the Long Days and Last Months, but once the Departing is bed-bound, the soles of her feet may be very sensitive to the least touch, or his ankles liable to →bedsores if he has a habit of sleeping with one foot crossed over the other. (→Nurses, physical therapists, and →hospice workers place cushions around the legs and ankles in such a way as to discourage leg-crossing, but lifelong habits return in the middle of the night when no one is looking.)

If the Departing is awake, she may appreciate a slow, gentle, well-lubricated massage of her soles, while he may want you to work along the sides. As circulation of blood to the extremities decreases, the feet may be cold or more insensitive than usual, so make sure that your own →hands are warm and smooth. Always ask whether it feels better for you to work from the heel toward the toes or (as in most massage manuals) from toes toward the heel. Maintain an even pressure, so that if you are asked to be gentler or firmer you will know exactly what to do. A one-way motion from heel to toes, or from toes up the arch to the heel, is best. Never use a back-and-forth or sawing motion unless asked to do so. Do not be so timid that your touch tickles rather than calms. Do not attempt massage if you have long or jagged finger→nails: the pain caused by a slight cut on the sole of a foot, given the thinness of the skin, can be excruciating.

You too may need a foot rub, if you have been on your feet much of the day attending to the needs of the bedridden. When others ask how they can help you, do not hesitate to ask for a massage. During the →Last Days, a massage may be rather a necessity than a luxury. It only takes a few minutes.

The bedridden do not like being bedridden, whether or not they are resigned to it. So, under appropriate circumstances, when they have energy and wrist strength, you might ask them to massage *your* feet. This may sound like a boorish imposition, may sound ghoulishly selfish, but it can give them a sense of being in the loop, able to share in the circle of care.

Vice versa, amid the recuperative warmth of a massage, they may begin to weep, reminded of a lost independence. Continue with your ministrations, but a bit more slowly, honoring the life they led when they could stand on their own two feet.

FLOCCILLATION

Near the end, the Departing may pluck at their clothing or at invisible pieces of lint in the air. This is a reliable →sign of imminent departure.

While you are talking with the Departing, they will casually take thumb and index finger to a pleat or wrinkle, or to the hair on their arms, the back of a hand, something floating in front of their eyes. They appear to be grooming themselves, and the air around them, as if all must be made presentable.

They are calm, deft, and persistent as they do this. They often are unaware of exactly what they are doing, but they may go on with it for ten minutes at a time, or longer.

Their hands dance lightly along their bodies, or out into the space around them, graceful.

To those at the bedside, floccillation is endearing and disturbing. Endearing, because there is something warmly human about this grooming, if that's what it is. Disturbing, because it can seem mindlessly compulsive, and distracting. Is it a sign of mental disintegration? In trying to catch and hold onto the smallest, most invisible elements of the world, are they losing touch with it all, with you, with themselves?

The medical community has no good answers. Is it a symptom of neurological or neuro-optical decline? Of cognitive loss? Sometimes it appears also during →delirium, dementia, fever, or exhaustion, but it is more predictable near death.

Floccillation summons metaphor, allegory. Why do people return to the preciously finite when faced with the infinite? To the particular and particulate, when faced with universals? {→Details} Do the Departing grab at invisible pieces of lint because that is all they can possibly do, any more, to put the world in order?

What if the plucking has nothing to do with grooming or organizing? What if it is a zen koan, a riddle of existence? Then again, in moments of great fatigue or long →waiting, don't we all tend to check for lint, or strands of hair, or spots on our clothes, almost without thinking, and with no real interest in what we find? Do we do that to assure ourselves of our own bodily presence, our liveliness in the face of a suspended animation?

There is a poem or a dance here, waiting to happen.

FOOD

You might think that the most furious arguments at the bedside would have to do with religion or inheritance; more often they have to do with food. Debate over dietary regimens can be as heated as over heaven and hell, given that during Long Days and Last Months, food is a realm over which those in bed and those at the bedside can both claim to have some power independent of doctors and nurses.

Because food habits are powerful and food lore seductive, and because a good appetite is so welcome a sign of recovery, theories of eating may even conflict with theories of nutrition. Isn't it emotionally and calorifically better for a person who is seriously ill and losing weight to eat something appealing to them--a forkful of steak, a jelly doughnut--rather than unsalted broth. And didn't I just read that chicken soup, red peppers, megadoses of Vitamin D have been proven to improve appetite, reduce tumors, restore the immune system?

In the →Last Months and Weeks, it may be surprisingly difficult to shake well-learned concerns for heart-healthy, low-fat, organic, or natural foods. Although it seems logical at the end to abandon all fears of cholesterol, saturated fats, salt, and hydrogenated oils, those at the bedside may be stuck with a lingering sense that if only the Departing had kept to a proper diet (no "empty-calorie" soft drinks, no red meat, no deep-fried snacks...), the Last Days would not have come so soon.

Similar thinking haunts people who have been on one weight-loss diet after another. Even as the end approaches, they tend to look at food in terms of calories and fat. At the extreme, I have known an anorexic teenager in the ER, near death, who kept asking about the calories in her IV drip.

Nutritional science itself is often bemused or contradictory when it comes to diets apt to specific conditions. Among all the vitamins, minerals, enzymes, and herbs on the shelves of health emporia, which is best for neuropathy? {→Pain II} How many have the courage to recommend marinol or marijuana brownies when all else fails to deal with pain? Uh oh, I smell another furious argument. Better calm down with Vitamin E to combat electron-hungry free radicals. Calm, you say?. . .

In hospital, everyone jokes about and deplores the food, but trust me, it's getting better, with more menu options. Still, at the end, you may want to bring in something delectable, if only for the aroma. But nothing greasy, for the aroma of grease lingers and begins to smell like death.

FORGETFULNESS

Write things down.

Write down the dates, times, and addresses of appointments. Write down the phone numbers and addresses of physicians, pharmacies, urgent care centers, ERs, hospitals, imaging centers, infusion centers, and medical supply companies. Write down the contact information of close friends, relatives, and neighbors, of visiting nurses, home health aides, caregivers and their agencies. Write down all medicines by name, dosage, times each day, and whether to be taken with or without food. Write down diagnoses and prognoses and keep track of dates of surgeries or biopsies, hospitalizations {→History, Part II}.

Hard copy is important. Do not trust exclusively to files on your computer, laptop, ipad, or smartphone, because all of the appropriate people may not know your passwords, or at the moment of greatest need the electronics may fail, batteries may be low, screens go wacky. If you rely on e-intelligence, update your files each day and e-mail them regularly to other caregivers and family.

Put all medical and lab appointments, home nursing visits, and planned excursions onto a large →calendar hung where everyone can see it. This is extra work, but invaluable.

If you pride yourself in having an unerring memory, more power to you. But you won't be available every hour, every day. Others, including those abed, will need quick access to what you know about appointments, medicines, visits, etc.

Besides, people under stress forget. People in a hurry forget. People who are trying to do five things at once forget. People with headaches forget. People who are tired forget. Unless superhuman, at the bedside you will also inevitably forget.

You are not experiencing the onset of early senility. You are →anxious, tired, besieged, and you just plain forgot. So, write things down, for yourself and for others.

And you thought this would be about Alzheimer's. Or the fog of chemo and painkillers. Or the missing names in last testaments. Or long-lost cousins. Or the passage of time.

I guess that you could say that this is a chapter about the passage of time. How, while stressed or beset, you may forget something probably important that a physician or nurse or aide or lawyer or who was it just told you a moment ago, or was it Tuesday?

So, write things down.

FRAMING

Everybody wants to help you understand what is going on, or asks you to help them understand. Throughout the Long Days and into the Last Days, there are tugs of war over context. Hoping to be helpful or to demonstrate a stoicism in the face of death, →physicians, →social workers, →case managers, and →friends will frame the situation for those at the bedside, sweetly or harshly, ethically or spiritually, medically or psychologically. And you too, you may feel the impulse to frame the situation for the Departing, and each day at the bedside to draw a bigger, or more detailed, picture of how things are.

Framing may be a comfort or may lead to a commandeering of experience and a co-opting of meaning. We constantly frame the world and its events for our children; as adults we tend to feel juvenalized, not rejuvenated, when others insistently frame the world for us. Not only those at the bedside but the Departing themselves deserve to be allowed to frame their own lives, concurrently and in retrospect, and to frame their deaths, in immediate prospect.

You need not agree with all the rest around the bedside about what a death means or a life meant: no need here for a majority opinion.

Best to let the framing become a way of seeing rather than a way of tidying up. In galleries as at deathbeds, the best frames for portraits encourage you to look again, and again, and again, at a person you thought was utterly familiar: a favorite, a friend, a lover, a father.

It is not that death estranges but that framing changes. Let it.

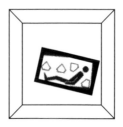

FRANKNESS

Today it is harder to talk about death than it was two hundred years ago, when mortality rates were so much higher, when almost every child experienced the death of a brother, sister, or parent, and when death occurred more often at home or on the battlefield than in hospital.

Over the last decades, medical schools have begun teaching future doctors how to speak about an approaching death, due in some measure to the influence of the hospice movement, in larger measure to new surgical procedures and drugs that extend life without affording a full rebound, so there are more people whose departures can be well anticipated and must be sanely discussed.

Few of us are prepared to speak plainly about death. And the less you have been at the bedside of the Departing during the Long Days, the less you can be certain of the degree of frankness that would be welcome during the Last Days. Certainly no one wants to be deceived with false assurances that death is a long way off when everyone outside the room knows different {→ETD.} Yet, a preternatural mournfulness at the bedside may appear to the Departing to be a form of upstaging: you who are obviously inconsolable must be deserving of more sympathy for your loss than the Departing for her departure. {→Grieving}

So there are three aspects to the problem of frankness:
1. how much to speak of death to the Departing;
2. how much to tell the youngest members of family. (→Young People)
3. how much to say about your own feelings, and with whom.

To be frank, in all three cases frankness is overrated. Not because honesty is harmful, but because the departure itself may not be uppermost in anyone's mind. For example (#1), the Departing may know full well that he is departing but ask you instead for an enthusiastic account of what makes you feel most alive. Or (#2), children may want to know more about what is planned for them, and who will be around, than details about the departure. Or (#3), you may have such mixed feelings of despair and relief that you cannot be frank without also becoming upset at your own ambivalence, and the Departing is in no state to serve as your counselor.

Little about the Last Days is absolutely straightforward.

FRIENDS

At the bedside, especially during the Last Days, family tend to take precedence over friends. Even over the closest of friends, lifelong friends. Families may know less about the life, fears, and philosophy of the Departing than do close friends, but there is a prevailing presumption that family, however out of touch or out of joint with the Departing, ultimately mean more than friends. Friends are sometimes not admitted into emergency rooms, →ICUs, or certain hospital wards where family have easy access, and medical staff are reluctant to share information with people who are "just friends." After all, family members have papers and cards that certify their relationship; we have few such papers or cards to define or certify friendships. A friend may be given →power of attorney for health care or even for finances, but a friend without such powers is, in the view of many institutions, no better than a stranger. So much for friends.

At home at the bedside, spouses, parents, or children may become jealous of friends who have a deeper connection with the Departing than they do, or who are more warmly welcomed. "Family friends" may be an exception, where they have strong cross-generational connections.

It is a hard thing to balance the standing of a →brother, sister, aunt, or uncle over against that of friends made and kept by the Departing in years lived separately from family. On the one hand, the Last Days are the last chances for the estranged to reconnect, for distant cousins to gather, for family feuds to be resolved, for the extended family to stretch its protective arms around all who have the slightest blood claim. On the other hand, the Last Days are the last chances for good friends to say their goodbyes, which cannot be brief or trite or smoothed over by commonplaces.

A balance must be reached that honors the Departing by honoring all whom the Departing has embraced, and still embraces. Yes, old friends can fade away, as can memories of grandparents or second cousins. And yes, each of us has widening gyres of friends, some close and constant, some rather acquaintances than helpmeets, as each of us has circles of relatives, some close to the bone, some barely tangible.

When the time comes, who should be at your bedside?

FUNERAL ARRANGEMENTS

Do you know families who have had funerals in their parlors and burials up the road apiece in the graveyard among eight prior generations? Most of us bury our dead among strangers and pay other strangers to arrange the service, then speak our eulogies in generic halls or mortuary chapels. A familiar face (a good friend, rabbi, minister, mullah, monk) may conduct the ceremony, but not always.

More and more people are paying for interments "pre-need," a disconcerting term that once referred simply to investing in a family plot. Today it refers to paying a mortuary or cremation* service up front for eventual retrieval and preparation of the body, for a casket and the cutting of a stone, or for cremation and an urn. Burial societies make the process simpler and less expensive, although membership does not preclude a higher price at time of need, or a long list of extras.

This can seem downright macabre, but it can be of comfort to those at the bedside, who will have at hand the best numbers to call and assurance that awkward details will be taken care of. It is when nothing at all has been arranged beforehand, as with the sudden death of a young person, that mortuary directors can prey on the disorientation of survivors to run up expenses by guiding them toward expensive caskets {→Plain Pine Boxes} and extras to which only royalty give any thought.

What is a funeral supposed to do? Consolidate the family? Reconcile family and friends? Mark the end of a bodily life while signaling the start of life on another plane? Confront tragedy and comfort the →grieving? Release everyone from the →ghosts of a familial past? Celebrate a life well lived?

Discuss this with the Departing. According to the answers, a funeral can change as mightily in tenor as in protocol. Aside from aspects of burial/cremation, no element in a funeral ceremony is established by law, although scripture and religious custom hold to the degree that one is observant.

There can be a funeral and a memorial, or one and not the other. A funeral comes first among traditions where burial is prescribed soon after death. A memorial can take place at anytime, anywhere.

The departure and the funeral or memorial will remain an indelible anniversary in your life; do not give it short shrift.

*Jewish, Islamic, and Eastern Orthodox Christian traditions forbid cremation.

GATEKEEPING

Gatekeeping may fall to you, or to anyone at the bedside for long stretches. You may not want the job, but you will need to protect the bedside from people who do not belong there and, usually, from →crowds.

Early on, consult the seriously ill and the Departing as to who is welcome. The list of the unwelcome may shock or sadden you; it may include members of the family, former lovers, and people claiming to be old friends or abandoned children. All such exclusions take precedence over your own sentiments.

When people learn that they are on the list of the unwelcome, they will direct their rage at you, not at the Departing. They may call you names, threaten legal action, appeal to other friends or family. Being excluded from a deathbed is often felt as more mean-spirited than exclusion from a wedding, since it is a last chance to make amends, forge a reconciliation.

Gatekeeping is too often honored in the breach. Who among us does not deserve another chance? People change: in the Last Days old feuds may be resolved and old grudges forgiven, may they not? Drawing up the initial List, the Departing may not have been of a mind to rethink relationships, but now? So how can you, or anyone, be responsible for →absolute foreclosure?

Seductive arguments, those, appealing to our most romantic natures. The longer the Last Days last, the more it seems that there could be time to heal all wounds except death itself.

It's difficult to resist such a generous notion of dying. You must. There are people who can instantly sour a room, a day, a dying. If it is a choice between a soured departure and embittered survivors, well, survivors have time in which to grow out of their bitterness. The Departing have none.

Nor can you make exceptions for someone *you* like whom the Departing would rather not see. Dying rarely changes the arithmetic of relationships, and→friendships are never perfectly distributive. That is, you can't count on your own best friends to be congenial company for the Departing. At the bedside. the most selfless thing you can do is to persist in an earnest advocacy for the Departing. Does this mean that you must admit those of the Departing's friends whom you detest?

You may now understand why gatekeeping is most effective when a joint endeavor among several who are regularly at the bedside and talk with each other.

GENERATIONS:
"THAT TALK COMMON TO SNOW"

snow again off the lake--whitefish
snow, flakes of bone in the white wind
across their walk--and a falling into
anatomy, what the snow does best
on the plains.

even in bright down
N seems too thin for the snow--
what he should be at the very end
of winter, slow and unwound; not now--
and my father wants to hold him up
like a man holding a clutch of hangers
on the way back home from the cleaners
but he doesn't. N must do this distance
on his own: a prescription.

so instead
my father makes talk, that talk
common to snow--history, drifts,
old fires, smoke, blocks of summer ice
sold by the heft. N's hollow as tongs
but what my father's after is the steel pin
at the center, the principle--the way you held
them *open* to hold the block.

  spiders, N says;
reminded me of spiders.

      they turn, look back
at the thread of their steps in the snow,
then go on, pushing their way across the light
stretches of ice. N's arms hang straight
from his shoulders--he's lost their balance--
and my father late from his own hospitals
wants to grab hold, hold N out
like a grocer holding a chain scale
out away from his hips to weigh the almonds
as they did on the street in the old days
in the summer in Chicago--what summers!
what haggling from carts! what dancing
arms on shoulders!--
but he doesn't.
Who can take the measure of cousins?

      N stops
in the snow, waiting for breath, forty yards
from the porch. what we've come to, H,
he says: a pretty pass: old men.

      nonsense,
my father says; the evil eye, and almost
takes him in his arms like a man
holding a woman in the cold--
as if love were a matter of weather--
but he doesn't. maybe, he says
to himself, if he slips, but not now.
we're only sixty, it's not time.

    the snow
comes to the black tops of their boots,
rides with them at each step. slow
going, N says and bends over, hands at knees,
to breathe.
my father wants to hold him
like a man holding a nest of buckets
above the snow--but he doesn't, says instead
we'll make it, both of us.

      at the porch steps
N slips and my father catches him
but N's so light my father stumbles
at the surprise and now both are lying
in the snow, two blue fish bright with down.
damn, N says, what a way to go.
and my father knows he will never hold him.

That was then. We circle up Mt. Palomar now
toward the dome, the telescope.
late October again, my father's smiling
at California sycamore, the maple out here.
Seasons, he says; they say there's snow
near the top.

And there is--an inch or two,
someone's lost linen, a Monday wash
blown off the line onto the slopes,
nothing permanent. I told N there was snow,
my father says, if you looked for it.

We're in the snow now in sneakers,
slipping and sliding. Stuff's real enough,
my father says. He's looking up and across
to the white meadows above us.
I want to hold him like a father
holding a son, show him the Rockies,
the High Sierras with their fields of ice
but I never will, he will never
let me. Real enough, I say; as real
as it gets. Stand right there, he says,
and he snaps a picture of me holding
still.

GHOSTS AND PHANTOMS

As the Departing become ghosts of themselves, they may see angels or ancestors or lost children. This can happen even with the resolutely secular or skeptic--although the phantoms may afterwards be explained by a spectral neurophysiology: scatters of light energy darting across the retina, or hallucinogenic images prompted by opiates.

Meanwhile, those at the bedside may begin to see their charge as phantoms, as someones no longer there. No matter how much the Departing may struggle to be inobtrusive in their pain and undemanding in their most basic needs, they do not like to be given up for dead. They may wish to drift off quietly, but they do not want to be denied solidity.

They →hear well, so to be ignored in conversations between people in the room is particularly stinging. And although they may be trying to detach themselves from things of this world (don't press them on this: they hold tenaciously to small treasures→Details), they may become frightened or saddened by the premature detachment of those at the bedside.

Drifting off is something else. As they drift off into sleep or a kind of inward staring, you too may drift off, lose focus. This is almost inevitable. None of us can be infinitely alert. Drifting off is not the same as drifting away; the first is a sort of refreshment, the second a distancing.

Friends or relatives who have drifted away years ago may show up out of nowhere: another species of phantom peculiar to the Last Days. For the first minutes there is consternation. Who is this? Why is he here? What does she want? These phantoms may want a lot (forgiveness, blessings), but they do not expect a lot so are rarely disappointed. It is their lot to make cameo appearances and speak a few lines about unknown corners in the life of the Departing. Then they leave.

A different sort of phantom are neighborhood children who appear for an instant at the bedside to touch the wrist of the Departing, whom they had befriended, or who make their way in and out of the room, unseen, to leave a gift on a bed table. These are secret gifts that only the Departing will understand. (Remember that small treasure?).

In some cultures there is a tradition at death of draping the mirrors in the room or throughout the house so that the spirit of the Departing is not caught and imprisoned in the glass. {→Reflection.} But during the Last Days the room is full of phantoms, some of whom can always be trusted.

GRIEVING

Grief is neither an event nor an accomplishment; it is a process, as much spatial as temporal. To be bereft is to feel deeply not just a loss but an absence. Grief is a process of making one's peace with that absence, of learning to take that hole in your life into account without being sucked in. That hole starts opening up when the seriously ill can no longer be as active as they once were, no longer the equal partner in projects or travels, no longer the physical lover or the steady companion at play or at work. {→Sex; Wives, Husbands, and Lovers}

During the Last Days, you will already have begun to grieve. Grieving is not the same as surrendering; it is facing the facts of two lives, your own and the life of the Departing. If you spurn sadness as an unhealthy or unhelpful pessimism, you will have a harder time with bereavement because you will have so much catching up to do.

That said, no one can do your grieving for you. Bereavement counselors may help you recognize where you may be stuck in the process, but they cannot help you take the full measure, full embrace, of the absence. This you must do yourself.

In the Days After, you may feel at sea or undocked, unable to settle back into any routine or familiar berth. Your house and bed may seem empty, the car missing a passenger, your office too silent. But whatever it was that kept you at the bedside is not lost; that you carry with you, like an amulet.

Grief can go on too long. Bereavement counselors are, really, ghostbusters. They are there, alone or as leaders of groups, to help release people from hauntings and resolve the guilt, sleeplessness, and loss of orientation that ensue when a person is obsessed by/with the dead.

On the other side of the mirror, you may have done most of your grieving weeks before the departure, and in the Days After you may be relieved, smiling, ready to take on the world. Bereavement counselors will say that you are still grieving, but you need not lose any sleep over the fact that you are not losing any sleep. And you certainly need not feel guilty for not feeling guilty, or for not appearing to be overwhelmed by a death.

Ritual mourning helps with grief and ghostbusting {→Funeral Arrangements; Obituaries and Obsequies; Sitting.} The rest you handle in your own way. There is no right way.

GRUMPS

People who have been grumps most of their life or with everyone other than a favorite nephew or golden retriever, such people do not ordinarily become kinder or gentler when seriously ill or on the eve of departure.

They may sleep a good deal more, and you may find this a welcome relief from persnickety demands, fault-finding, back-handed compliments, all of which you have borne with an equanimity for which you deserve beatification. You may even have resisted temptations to give them another dose of→ *p.r.n.* sedatives or painkillers at the shortest safe interval so that they remain quiet and you too can get some sleep.

In the best of circumstances, with all the money in the world, obnoxious people do not get the best of care. Staff in hospital or →SNFs avoid them whenever possible, come reluctantly to their call lights. At home, neighbors stop visiting; hired help may quit after being harassed once too often. As a result, you will need more frequent →respite.

Unless a favorite nephew, you will feel ambivalent about caring for grumps. No doubt they've brought all their troubles on themselves (by smoking, drinking, or eating too much, by skipping meds and ignoring doctors, or by alienating friends who could have helped before it was too late). They're taking you away from people who worry that your own health is being sapped, your business suffering, your job in jeopardy, and for what? He'll never be grateful, she'll only demand more.

Of course, grumps are human too, and may have hearts of gold (or bank accounts used for →blackmail). Maybe they've been sick for years and they're not intrinsically grumpy, it's the sickness that made them grumpy.

There's the rub. The strain and pain of serious illness can indeed turn good people into grumps, and if not the illness, then long hospitalizations and/or the strain and pain of medical diagnostics and interventions (biopsies, surgeries, radiation, chemotherapies) and/or the side-effects of drugs.

But grumps take their toll, whatever the cause. You'll need to be on guard against compromising care out of spite, frustration, or anger. On guard, too, against elevating your own sense of "being used" into a crown of martyrdom. On guard, finally, against becoming a grump yourself, which can happen at the drop of a pin. Didn't you hear that? Why didn't you pick it up? What's wrong with you? I'll bet there's half a dozen pins on the floor waiting to give me tetanus. And what do you care?

HAIR

Whatever the setting, someone at the bedside always seems to be arranging the hair of the Departing, smoothing it back, pushing a strand to one side, adjusting a curl.

The bald sometimes escape these almost-automatic caresses, but few depart entirely bald. Those who do, who during the Long Days have undergone chemotherapy and radiation treatments, they have already adjusted to their loss of hair-- more adeptly and often more calmly than family or friends at the bedside, who may still hold dear a picture of the Departing from an earlier era, almost always with a full head of hair.

What is this obsession with hair, its neatness, its style, its gloss, its sheen? Is it our simplest way of making death presentable? Domesticating the wildness of death?

Or, since hair appears to continue to grow for a while after death, is our obsessive touching of it meant to reassure the Departing and ourselves of some continuity? Will the hair remember our caresses when the mind and body are gone?

Or do we have a need to assert some sort of personal order and flair during Last Days that are otherwise so irregular and unkempt, with →tubes dangling, bedclothes and pillows awry, complexion ghastly? Is this why some wives insist on shaving the cheeks and chins of their husbands during the Last Days?

Or is this fussing with hair our response to the acrobatics of Beauty and Truth in the face of a departure? Hair grows despite us, as if from some elemental root of ourselves, an inadvertent but consistent expression of our liveliness, our genetics, our roots. And we reach out to caress the remaining strands as if to hold for a moment what otherwise cannot be held, the truth of what is irrepressible in us. Which is, one could argue, what is beautiful about us. And true.

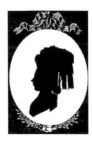

HANDS AND GLOVES

Watch their hands. They flutter, pick, open, release, smooth out the sheets. For those trained in end-of-life care, the hands talk when the Departing do not. Fisted up or pressing into a coverlet, they speak of →anxiety or →pain; open and loose, they speak of rest. Reaching, fluttering, they speak of hallucination or restlessness. Curling in or covering the genitals or throat, they speak of a sense of loss or fear.
{Also→Floccillation; Signs.}

Hold their hands. Throughout the Long Days and into the Last Days, they will hold your hands, sometimes with a fierceness you have not experienced since childhood. Even people who lifelong have been undemonstrative, who do not hug their family or touch friends with those light taps that mean "it's good to be here with you," even they will hold hands near the end, return your touch.

Wash their hands. Sensations of griminess or coldness or roughness may afflict them, though they say nothing. Use a warm soft washcloth, slightly wet.

Apply lotion. The hands, particularly the spaces between the fingers, may become dry and red. Massage the hands gently with a non-perfumed lotion. Do not use alcohol swabs, towelettes, or alcohol-based cloths that dry out the skin.

Now about gloves. As late as the 1960s, some women wore gloves whenever they went out, to protect their hands (and finger→nails) from an impure world. Gloves as formal wear have all but vanished; gloves as protection against a dangerous world have returned with a vengeance not only for physicians, nurses, dentists, and dental hygienists, but for postal workers, airplane stewards, and janitors.

Should you be wearing gloves when helping feed, change, dress, or bathe the ill or Departing? Probably not. Gloves are necessary only when they have
--highly sensitive skin (e.g., from certain allergies or type 2 diabetes);
--ulcers or other skin afflictions or wounds that are exuding pus and serous fluids;
--tender lesions (e.g., from a compromised immune system, burns, or →bedsores);
--an infectious disease that can be transmitted by touch.

HANDS AND GLOVES, continued

If you must use gloves, you will have choices to make: size (small, medium, large); latex or nitrile/vinyl; powdered (or lightly powdered, or powder free, or coated with aloe); flat cuff, beaded, or rolled; scented or unscented; textured or smooth. Since you will be using and discarding gloves more often than you would imagine, purchase them in bulk according to your budget. Unless circumstances otherwise dictate, opt for non allergenic (non-latex) gloves in a size that slips on easily and fits snugly without tearing. Lightly powdered or coated gloves slip on most easily but are more expensive, as are cuffed or textured gloves.

To handle someone with (kid) gloves is literally off-putting: the sick and the Departing will suspect that they are being treated as "untouchables." Unless there is a medical imperative, the uncloaked touch of your hands is ever to be preferred, even when the Departing has itchy skin from jaundice, common during the Last Days. Who would wish the last warm touches of a hand to be five-finger exercises in synthetic blue or green?

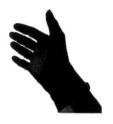

HAVE YOU THOUGHT OF...

Question: Have you thought of contacting the American _____[*put disease here*] Society?
Answer: They sent me some brochures and advice on how to put them into the will.
Answer you'd like to make: You think I'm an idiot? They were first on my list.

Question: Have you considered the _____[*put religion or profession here*] rest homes?
Answer: That just didn't work out.
Answer you'd like to make: You think that I didn't spend weekend after weekend checking out every place within two hundred miles of here? You think I didn't calculate down to the dime the family's resources and call a dozen →agencies to get some help with insurance details? Do you honestly think the Departing would be happy in one of those places? Would you like to be shoved into one of those places?

Question: Have you tried acupuncture or _____[*put other non-Western therapy here*]?
Answer: Yes.
Answer you'd like to make: You think I wouldn't look for relief for the Departing in any corner I could find it? And just what kind of doctor are you?

Question: What about nutrition therapy? My daughter in medical school is big on anti-oxidants and _____[*name your essential vitamin, mineral, or....*]
Answer: It worked for a while.
Answer you'd like to make: **** it, he can't even swallow, she has difficulty keeping anything down, we've asked for all IVs to be disconnected, and you're talking about vitamins? {→Food}

Question: Did you call →social services or _____[*insert other public agency here*]?
Answer: They got us this commode.
Answer you'd like to make: Have you ever been run to the ground by people whom you've just met who think they know exactly who you are, what you need, what must be done, and what your responsibilities are to *them*?

HAVE YOU THOUGHT OF..., on and on

Question: Would you like me to follow up on those
_____[*put leads here*] I gave you last week?
Answer: Thanks, but it's time to let go. I know you're trying to help, but....
Answer you'd like to make: Get off my back! I've done everything that could be done, and some things that really couldn't, and I'm sick and tired of everyone insinuating that I've been lazy or stupid or stingy or cold.

Question to yourself: Why do the most well-meaning of →friends and relatives make such persistently obnoxious suggestions?
Answer: Because they are well-meaning and cannot possibly know all that you have tried. Because they do not know the Departing as well as you do. Because they have not gone through all the →stages of expectation and disappointment that you have gone through with the Departing, so they cannot possibly appreciate your anger with questions that to them seem innocently helpful.

Question: What can I do for you?
Answer: Make me dinner.

HEARING / VOICES

Generally, hearing is the last of the senses to go. This means that the Departing will be able to hear you until near the end. They may not look like they can hear you, and they may not be able to respond, but they can hear you. Not only your words but your tone of voice will register.

So: Never speak to others in the room as if the Departing were not present. I repeat: Never speak to others in the room as if the Departing were not present.

The Departing may also, while on certain medications, hear voices and sounds that you cannot. Such voices and sounds may be aural hallucinations. Or they may be tinnitus, an intermittent (or intermittently obnoxious) noise in the ears that can resemble ocean waves, the whistle of a tea kettle, or the screech of brakes. If the Departing still sports powerful hearing aids, they may be the awful screeks of electrical interference.

All of which means that you cannot presume to be hearing *for* the Departing. She can hear for herself. You may be able to help him hear better by getting drugs switched or hearing aid batteries replaced. It's tough to eliminate tinnitus, whose origins are disputed and for which there is no known short-term therapy. However, since tinnitus may be exacerbated by waxy plugs in the ears, by aspirin, quinine, streptomycin, and some opiates, and by temporo-mandibular joint (TMJ) problems, you may be able to help reduce tinnitus--but act only at the request of the Departing. Those who have lived with tinnitus for years and tried dozens of "cures" may not want to subject themselves to more experiments. For those to whom tinnitus is a new and disturbing experience, efforts toward palliation can be useful, especially if these require only a change of prescriptions or an ear cleaning. TMJ problems can be helped substantially by craniosacral massage at the bedside.

You may also find yourself listening closely to the voice and breath of the Departing so as not to miss a barely-spoken word. Whether or not you realize it, you will also be listening for signs of the nearness of departure--a weakening voice, a deepening rattle in the throat, more erratic breathing {→Last Breaths; Aspiration}. Your ears will then begin to play tricks on you, and you may become intently aware of the sound of your own breathing (from which can come, on occasion, a mild panic attack, so leave the room for a while and settle down).

Everyone, of course, is listening for the →Last Words.

HELP (at home)

Remember, you cannot do this alone. You should not. For your sake and for the sake of the seriously ill and Departing, you need help during Long Days and into the Last Days. You are no less of a person for seeking, and accepting, help.

You need not accept all offers or be hemmed in by helpers, but you must realize that dying is not dyadic: more than two are usually involved. That is a good thing.

This chapter is not about →selfishness, not about keeping the Departing to yourself. It's about stubborn independence. Pride. Privacy. Out of pride or shame or a desperate desire to appear autonomous, the Departing may ask that only you stay at the bedside, only you change the bedding, only you administer the drugs, only you prepare the food, only you do the shopping, only you change the dressings, only you sort the mail, only you rearrange the pillows, only you . . . .

Once upon a time all this might have been possible. It is not possible during the →Last Months, let alone during the Last Days. You need help. If you do not get help, you will get a bad cold, sprain an ankle, throw your back out, strain a shoulder, or lose so much →sleep that you begin to misplace things--a wallet or purse, a cell phone, eyeglasses, a key ring, an address book you had a minute ago, it was right there in your hands.

The Departing is not entirely in your hands. In most cases there will be nurses and home health aides coming in, friends and relatives phoning or stopping by. Granted, it may all get to be too much, and you may wish for some quiet, some time alone, hours apart from the strange hurly-burly and →grumpiness that often surrounds the bedside. {→Gatekeeping.}

In the long run, however, you need sturdy help. You and the Departing can still make the basic decisions and determine the tenor of care. You just plain need help: perhaps in →turning or lifting the body abed, or cleaning up, or finding a way to stop a neighbor's dog from yapping. Accepting help does not mean that you are irresponsible, incompetent, or weak. It means that you accept the fact that you are part of a wider human community in which illness and death are common, and where helping at the bedside is a collective enterprise.

Do not worry about crying wolf. During →emergencies and →acute episodes you have people to call. When there is no "real" emergency, during Long Days, help for any reason may be a great relief. You may simply need someone to give you permission to sit down elsewhere than at the bedside.

HIPAA (pronounced "Hippa")

Health Insurance Portability and Accountability Act of 1996, that is. You can read all about it at www.hhs.gov/ocr/privacy/, but here's the gist: anyone who wants to obtain another's medical or hospital records, or to communicate with another's health providers about anything other than scheduling, or to sit in on medical consults must have explicit permission from the patient. (The rule may be waived when a patient is unconscious or unavailable and health providers need quickly to relay information to family or →caregivers.)

"Health providers" includes physicians, nurses, hospital staff, skilled nursing and assisted living or board-and-care staff, hospice staff, dialysis and infusion technicians, physical therapists, social workers, psychologists, pharmacists, etc.

In practice, this means that whether you are a spouse, a parent, a child, a relation, a close friend, a lover, or someone with →power of attorney, you are likely to be required by health providers to have the person in question sign a form granting you access to health-related information and status as someone with whom they have permission to speak about medical issues. If you are actively involved in someone else's care, you will therefore need to ask about such forms, and have them signed, at every physician's office, hospital, nursing facility, infusion or dialysis center, rehab center, health insurance company, etc.

HIPAA does allow you to pick up another's prescriptions, medical supplies, →x-rays, lab results and so forth without written permission, though you will have to sign for them.

HIPAA allows a person to deny access to *anyone*--a spouse, parent, child, ex, etc.

HIPAA declares that each person has a right to see and get a copy of all of his/her health records, although a form for release of such records may have to be signed for each separate stay at a medical facility. Everyone has a right to amend or protest information on those records. If these rights are denied, there is a set-up for filing complaints and getting them resolved.

But beware. The following need not comply with HIPAA: life insurance and workers compensation carriers, school districts, employers, child protective service agencies, and many law enforcement agencies. They may ask for signed HIPAA forms but are not obliged to follow HIPAA regulations, so medical privacy is not assured when filling out their forms, etc.

As you might expect from all the etceteras, see →Paperwork.

HISTORY, Part I: Biographical

Regrets, regrets . . . one of the most common regrets of the →Last Days has to do, paradoxically, with history. You regret that months earlier, during the Long Days or Last Months, when the Departing was perfectly coherent and eager to talk, you did not take down his philosophy of life, record her story, videotape him on his morning walk, photograph her at that wooden bench overlooking the ocean. Now you are stuck with what each person at the bedside remembers, and with whatever the Departing chooses fragmentarily to recall.

If the Departing is at →home, some of the rooms have probably been rearranged to accommodate a hospital bed and medical paraphernalia. Even so, you can take pictures of each room, of the paintings on the walls, the books on the shelves, the view from the windows. And you can shoot still photographs or digital video of the Departing in moments of lucidity holding court or a cup of water.

But as the Last Days progress, as skin pales and faces grow gaunt, cameras seem out of place. A small digital voice recorder can be more inconspicuous and ready to go at a moment's notice when meaningful conversations start up, or when you are being briefed by a nurse or a physician. In hospital or other medical facilities, there are more echoes and disturbances, so voice recorders will have to cope with a good deal of background →noise.

If you are becoming suspicious of the care being given, or of the diagnoses and treatments, you may also want to record bedside consultations with physicians, and physical therapists, so that later you can go over the details of the conversation.

Such recording is useful whether or not you are worried about the quality of care, the logic behind a diagnostic procedure, or the reasoning behind a prognosis. Since neither patients nor their partners easily or fully register all of the information and implications of what is said at meetings with physicians or social workers, it is best to make audio recordings of these meetings, whether in emergency rooms, hospitals, skilled nursing facilities, dialysis units, rehab gyms, or doctors' offices. And do ask for copies of all lab reports, medical progress charts, and scans, with their accompanying readings or interpretations.

Which brings us to→History, Part II, Medical.

HISTORY, Part II: Medical

As an historian of medicine and a case manager, I must take note of a second sort of history: the medical history.

From earliest times, medical histories were dialogues. Patients talked about what had been happening to them and what they felt to be wrong; doctors inquired about their temperaments, their physical and mental constitution, origins and symptoms of their complaints, and what they had already tried by way of cure. West and East, astrological signs and portents as well as networks of kin were part of this work-up, and in some places still are. But in modern times, medical histories have become more extensive rather in terms of allergies, scans, implanted devices and genetic factors than movements in the heavens.

From well before the Long Days and well into the Last Weeks, a medical history will be taken orally by ER physicians, by hospitalists and the specialists they call in, regardless of what has already been presented five days, hours, or minutes ago, as if no one trusts anyone else and certainly not the patient.

Doctors may consult existing records, paper or electronic, but they will insist on running verbally through their own →checklist of questions in order to create (anew) a medical history.

Everywhere, in medical and even in dental offices, the patient will already have been required to fill out forms detailing current medications; allergies; →pre-existing conditions and today's complaints; prior illnesses, hospitalizations, surgeries, and diseases that may run in the family.

This is frustrating, eventually maddening. You just spent twenty-five minutes helping check off box after box on six pages of an omnibus form, so why is the nurse or doctor now asking the same questions again? If every form-filling session is going to be followed up by an oral interrogation, why bother with any of the →paperwork?

The solution is to create (digitally, if possible) a medical history and list of medications, and to update these each week. Make hard copies and bring these to all medical settings, where you can ask the staff to photocopy them for their files. Then, when and wherever you encounter an omnibus form, you can simply insert an asterisk referring to the medical history that you have supplied on the attached sheets.

Format as follows on next page:

HISTORY, Part II: Medical, continued

<u>First Page</u>:

Medical History, updated __/__/___, prepared by _____

for **N A M E** and birthdate __/__/____
Social Security Number, if patient OKs (=Medicare #, often)

Known allergies (prior life-threatening reactions to drugs, bee stings, nuts, shellfish, red wine, perfume...)
Implanted **devices** (ports, pain pumps, pacemaker, by brand)

Medical Insurance Policy Names, ID + Group Numbers
Prescription Drug Program

Home address
Home phone + cell numbers
Emergency contacts (2-3): Name, Relationship, Phone
Physicians: Contact Info for Primary + specialists

Current diagnoses (i.e., carcinoma, asthma, renal failure...)
Current Medications
--Prescription drugs by name/generic, dosage, purpose
--Over-the-Counter supplements, vitamins, minerals, etc.

<u>Second Page:</u>

Medical History continued, page 2,

N A M E and birthdate

Family History of [colon cancer, heart attack, stroke...]

Ongoing Therapies
Physical/Occupational, with whom and how often?
Psychological/Psychiatric, with whom? (if patient approves)

Hospitalizations and Procedures
List most recent first, with brief account of reasons/results:
All Surgeries, by date, including implantation of devices
Hospitalizations, by date, place, reason (last 2-3 years)
Scans: x-rays, ultrasound, CT, PET, MRI (last 12 months)
Most significant chemistries: blood tests, urine/kidney , etc.
(last 12 months)

HOLDING ON

The stories are legion: people holding on, against the odds, to reach an historic marker or →anniversary. Dying upon reaching a 99th birthday, not weeks before. Dying only after a certain grandchild or estranged spouse or long-lost sister has paid a call. Dying, in other words, when it is a good day to die. {→Buying Time; ETD; Last Breaths}

The stories are legion: people struggling for breath and words so long as they believe that someone at or near the bedside desperately needs them. Holding on as a way of holding others steady: the courage of the dying on behalf of those who will be living on.

The stories are legion: people waiting for everyone to leave-- out-of-state visitors all gone, loved ones asleep, attendants drowsing--in order to die alone, no one to hold them back, no one to make a fuss, no one to call for help. A quiet exit.

Do the Departing hold on because they love life or because they love you? Do you hold onto them because they don't deserve to die (so young / this way), or because you need them for yourself? {→Selfishness}

Imagine the Last Days as a wrestling match in reverse: you win not by going to the mat but by touching each other ever more softly; not by an assiduous pinning down but by a deft and touching release.

HOME

Does anyone *not* want to be at home during Long Days and Last Days? I can think of some instances: too much noise at home or in the vicinity; pushy neighbors; reminders of bad times; rooms too cramped for a comfortable "hospital" bed; too many steps up to a bathroom or bedroom; an ailing spouse; a high crime area; civil war.

Let me continue to be contrarian. What does it matter where one is during the →Last Months and Days, if these are going to be spent in bed, looking inward, communing with family and friends, or asleep under the heavy impress of →pain drugs and soporifics? What's all the (→hospice) fuss about dying at home? Isn't the desire for a death at home as anachronistic, say, as the pride once taken in people "dying with their boots on"?

Home. In mobilized industrial societies, it's unlikely that a person will die in the same house where he was born, in the same town where she grew up, or even in the same county or state. And "seniors" will already have moved to smaller digs, especially if they have lost a spouse. So what's all this sentiment about home?

What's wrong, therefore, with nursing homes, retirement homes, homes for the →ageing and elderly? Isn't home where the hearth is?

I write this not because I find these contrarian arguments entirely credible but because you will have moments at the bedside when you desperately want to go home, to be back in your own bed or at your own desk. Then it will strike you that the Departing is not just leaving but leaving *home*. And although many faiths promise new homes in peculiarly earth-like heavens, you will begin to think about your current home in a new light. What's at home that's not here? How can you make the Departing "feel at home" in his new hospital bed? In her new community of the memory-less and immobile?

A collection of ceramic frogs? A hand-knitted coverlet? A painting by a grandchild? A photo album? A digital photo album?

Home. Exactly what is that? And where?

HOSPICE (<Latin *hospes*, to host a guest)

Decades after the advent of the modern Hospice Movement in 1967, hospitals and nursing homes still had wings for the terminally ill. These were open wards, patrolled rather for quiet and cleanliness than for medical care. Painkillers were doled out meagerly, as nurses and doctors had been taught to fear addiction more than shrieking. The wealthy, as they had done for centuries, passed their Last Days at home, attended by private physicians and nurses less stingy with analgesics.

Under the influence of Cicely Saunders, a former nurse, a medical social worker, and then a physician who founded St. Christopher's Hospice in one of the poorer areas of London, hospitals and doctors began to reconsider their approaches to the →Last Days. Some charitable institutions for the care of dying patients, also called hospices, had been founded earlier by orders of nuns in Lyon (1842), Dublin (1879), and London (1905). The new movement was inspired by David Tasma, a terminal cancer patient whom Saunders met in 1948 and who left funds toward the establishment of a place where, instead of being warehoused, the dying were granted respect, privacy and, as much as medically possible, freedom from pain.

In the United Kingdom and Canada, hospice care was linked with National Health programs whose support teams worked with the dying in hospitals and at home; in Québec, a different term was adopted: "palliative care" (*soins palliatifs*). In the U.S., the Hospice Movement began in 1974 in New Haven as a not-for-profit agency which, at little or no cost to clients, took over care once a person left the hospital to spend the Last Days at home. Nine years later, the Medicare Hospice Benefit was implemented, leading to a proliferation of hospices that work with people in hospitals, at home, or at their own in-patient facilities.

This background is key to understanding hospice services and ambitions. Hospice programs mean to be conscientiously comprehensive but also insist on certain protocols. The Medicare Hospice Benefit (through which most U.S. hospices work) requires an official prognosis of death within six months, as determined usually by a primary physician, but it can be renewed for additional six-month periods where a person lives on with the same or other perilous, irremediable conditions. There must be no ongoing treatment other than what is considered palliative.

HOSPICE. continued

Medicare requires visits from →social workers, so they are part of all hospice teams, which include nurses, physicians, and home health aides. A hospice may also require that there be 24-hour attendance upon the Departing at home, but no hospice supplies nurse's aides or home care for more than a few hours a week {but see also →Respite.}.

For people with limited bank accounts, hospice benefits are substantial: an ambulance from the hospital or nursing home to a hospice facility or back home; hospital beds; all medications and skin care products; tanks of →oxygen, →pain pumps, commodes, and diapers. And although a hospice's beds (in its own facility or part of another) are usually restricted to those with an →ETD of a week or less, hospice groups do not expect all of their clients to pass swiftly, so will work with other agencies in the longer run.

At any time, a person contracted with a hospice group can opt out on twenty-four hours notice.

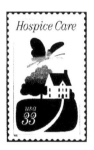

HOT & COLD

Fever, once considered a disease, has been demoted to a symptom. But during the Last Days, when so much of the body's preparation for departure is going on invisibly, under cover of sleep, signs of a fever may be peculiarly welcome. Something can usually be done for a fever, and those at the bedside can feel useful as they pass a cool cloth over the forehead of the Departing, gently around the ears and neck.

During the Long Days as well as the Last Weeks, nurses and physicians may advise administering acetaminophen (Tylenol, etc.) for comfort's sake, or something stronger when a fever is high (over 102 F). Fevers come and go during the Last Weeks and do not tell you anything about the nearness of a departure.

With fever there is sweating; bedsheets will need changing. {→Bedsores, Laundry.} With fever there is →thirst; water pitchers will need filling. With fever there is often a sensitivity to intense →light; shades will need to be drawn, lamps lowered or redirected. With fever there may be chills and trembling, for which sheets, →blankets, and pillows may need to be rearranged. How satisfying that there is so much to do.

Chills or not, the Departing will become cooler as metabolism slows and circulation in the arms and legs becomes sluggish. The arms and legs will begin to turn bluish, and the underside of the body (the skin between the shoulder blades and on either side of the spine, the rump, the backs of the legs) will darken. A blanket can help, but never a heating pad or an electric blanket, which are problematic: electrical proximity to an oxygen tank; too focused a heat; the fragility of the skin.

You may feel yourself becoming alternately hot or cold, flushed or numb. Long hours at the bedside can do this to anyone who has not had enough to eat or drink and not enough hours asleep and dreaming. If your body is losing its capacity to regulate its temperature, that's a clear and immediate sign that you need help, nourishment, and →respite.

As for emotional changes from hot to cold, from remorse to resentment, from love to withdrawal, or from passion to dispassion, these are to be expected. As the Departing withdraws from the living, the emotions of those at the bedside can run high and unpredictably. Better this than a steady, unconvincing lukewarmness. Steadiness during the Last Days may be an admirable quality, but it is not something to maintain at all costs, not something indisputably heroic We are all creatures of the sun and are borne along on a solar wind.

HYPOCHONDRIA

As you watch over someone with a terminal illness, you begin to suspect that you too are afflicted.

You are not.**

**With hypochondria, there are always asterisks. Hypochondria feeds on asterisks and small print.

* * * * *

Certain diseases, rare in industrialized countries, are so highly contagious and communicable that you should avoid contact with all secretions: bacterial meningitis, bubonic plague, Ebola virus, Hanta virus, hemorrhagic fevers, smallpox, typhoid fever.

Hepatitis (A, B, C, E) and HIV/AIDS are more common. Only hepatitis B is considered highly contagious, although C (like HIV/AIDS) can be transmitted by blood, by sharing of drug needles, and by unprotected intercourse. Carriers of A enjoy a normal life expectancy, as do carriers of B unless infected by two strains of the virus, or elderly and frail, or alcoholics, or immune-compromised by chemotherapy. Carriers of C usually develop chronic cirrhosis of the liver. Hepatitis E is contracted through drinking water contaminated by fecal matter; the genotype of E prevalent in developed countries rarely causes hepatitis outbreaks or deaths, most of which occur in East and South Asia.

HIV/AIDS qualifies as a pandemic, though mortality rates have declined since the advent of highly active antiretroviral therapy, or HAART

Tuberculosis (TB) is not highly contagious. Although *Mycobacterium tuberculosis* is easily spread through the air by coughing, sneezing, and spitting and a third of the world has been infected by the bacterium, most people have "latent TB," where one's lifetime risk of falling ill with TB is less than 10%--unless immune-compromised by malnutrition, diabetes, HIV, or heavy tobacco use. Even then, most forms of active TB other than those that are multi-drug-resistant are fully curable. Just to be safe, if you have had hours of close exposure to someone with active TB, you must get tuberculin PPD (purified protein derivative) skin tests to determine whether you have acquired the bacterium--the first test as soon as you learn of the exposure, the second test 8-12 weeks later, since there is an incubation period after exposure before PPD tests can show up positive.

Bottom line: At the bedside in the North America, Europe, Australia, and Japan, you need not worry about contagious diseases, except as noted above. When visiting people in isolation, observe all posted notices for wearing protective gowns and masks. The majority of people in isolation are there because they have compromised immune systems and can be easily infected by you, but some are in isolation because they are in the most contagious stage of a disease.

IATROGENESIS {→History, Part II; Lawyers}

Which means, harm caused by a physician or a prescribed drug, whether a life-threatening infection, a chronic disease, or death.

Which implies: rising rates of malpractice insurance and the reluctance of new MDs to enter general practice, where office fees are insufficient to meet the expense of such insurance.

Which leads to: legal disputes over limits of liability; policy debates over national health insurance; fury over the slowness of approval of new drugs or procedures.

Which redounds upon issues of →advocacy, medical intelligence, and power relations among patients, caregivers, →nurses, and →physicians. Consider Dr. House, who during sixty minutes of high television drama and high-end advertising, nearly kills each patient with costly, painful diagnostic procedures and non-standard uses of drugs while encouraging home invasions, and who almost always restores the patient to the community, with every prospect of many enjoyable years to come.

Hooey. Such rescues are vanishingly improbable, and make desperation the rationale for acceding to tyranny. Much more probable are cases in which physicians remain stumped about causes and try hectically to manage symptoms, all the while dubious of the capacity of a patient or anyone at the bedside to follow the logic of their course of treatment, especially when bloodwork, x-rays, and all scans fail to pinpoint a culprit.

But iatrogenesis is tricky. Staphylococcal infections (notably MRSA) from stays in hospital are the most notorious. Equally common in hospital are misreadings of doctor's orders and the misplacing of lab reports-- so you must be vigilant and vocal, asking supervisors to re-check orders and records or to contact physicians.

The more complex the situation, the more difficult it will be to prove significant harm caused by misstep or negligence. If you suspect iatrogenesis, mention this quietly to others at the bedside and begin to document it, but make no accusations unless the problem requires instant repair. Submit all →paperwork needed to obtain work-ups and notes, lab and scan results, procedure reports. →Question physicians about treatments, and do not hesitate to remark on contradictions or gaps in logic, all the while recording the conversation. Along the way, ask yourself: Is your own frustration, →sadness, or despair driving you to blame the medical world into which you have all been thrust, willy-nilly? Or is the issue clear?

IDENTITY

Who is that person in the bed?

You can't predict how much a serious illness, terrible pain--or a regime of potent drugs for managing both--may change a person, make her unrecognizable, him a stranger.

In hospitals and →SNFs, patients sport plastic bracelets printed with their names and birthdates, sometimes a second bracelet noting allergies or a →DNR. At home a similar bracelet is a good idea. Etched with name, emergency contacts, allergies, and chronic conditions, it is useful for 911 personnel, visiting RNs, and those who find a person wandering the streets.

Bracelets, of course, do not resolve the existential problem. Consider individuals suffering from a neurological disorder called Capgras Syndrome, who accuse all family and friends of being impostors because they do not look or sound *exactly* like the persons they remember: a wisp of hair is out of place, the voice foggy, the skin more freckled. Those at the bedside tend toward an obverse Capgras: given all that s/he has been going through, how can I talk to him as if he were the same? how can I be sure that she understands me as she always did? And if we do seem to be on a familiar wavelength, aren't we enacting a radio-pretence?

I would not worry. Yes, personality reversals do manifest after strokes (the shy may talk sexy or swear like sailors, world travelers may roar narrowly racist epithets). Yes, some drugs turn the angelic →grumpy, the articulate into sputtering fools. Yes, there is such a thing as "chemo-brain," a mental cloudiness that can result also from radiation treatment.

But soon enough that person you came to sit beside will be recognizable, intelligible, and demand to be heard as herself, as much as pain, drugs, disorientation, and a snoring →roommate will allow. (Except, sadly, for advanced Alzheimer's.)

What you should be more worried about is identity theft. The seriously ill and regularly hospitalized are vulnerable to identity theft because they have become used to giving out private information to medical offices, clinics, hospitals, insurance companies, pharmacists . . . and because one of their few remaining avenues of independence is to act on their own in positive response to intriguing e-mails or phone solicitations.

Ironic: that such desperate self-assertion at a time when one most wants to reclaim oneself should most compromise identity.

INTENSIVE CARE

Shouldn't all care be intensive care?

Is "intensive care" in contrast to extensive care? One gives intensive care for a short time, extensive care for the duration?

Or in contrast to relaxed care? Intensive care invokes constant surveillance by a focused team of specialized personnel, relaxed care a casual if regular monitoring by a nurse and an aide, with brief four-minute visits by physicians?

Or is it really a contrast between acute jeopardy and chronic danger? Intensive care staves off death at close quarters, while ordinary care deals with threats progressively more distant as a patient moves from hospital to →SNF to home.

Or is it a tremulous state of being, where one is on the knife's edge between life and death?

When you hear that "s/he's in Intensive Care," what are you supposed to think? Are you to be reassured that he's receiving a higher level of medical attention? Or terrified that she's in such peril that intensity is a necessity? Puzzled that what was to be a "typical" procedure entails a stay in medical limbo? Or upset at a derailment from the normal arc of recuperation?

Such tensions have prompted hospitals to refine their labels. Doesn't a Critical Care Unit (CCU) feel more reassuring than an Intensive Care Unit (ICU)? Doesn't it sound like progress to be moved from an ICU to a Progressive Care Unit (PCU) rather than a High-Dependency Unit (HDU)? Doesn't it sound more purposive to be sent to a Cardiac [Coronary] Intensive Care Unit (CICU) than to a general Intensive Treatment Unit (ITU)?

Whatever you call it--CCU, ICU, PCU--the unit is never identical to an Emergency Room (ER), where people must be stabilized and released, or hospitalized for further care.

ICU bedsides are more difficult and more restrictive. →Friends may not be admitted. Children may be excluded for fear of infection. Monitoring is so frequent and →tubing (for breathing, feeding, drainage, IV fluids) so all-enveloping that talk will be interrupted by nurses, by the beeps and buzzes of environing equipment, by the pumping of respirators or a tube down the throat. It may be hard to find a →hand to hold that is not beset by →needles, bandages, blisters.

Your presence, however, will still be registered. By ear; by sternum {→Breastbone}; by something so deep within us that "intensive" doesn't begin to explain it.

INVERSE CARE LAW

Julian Tudor Hart wrote an essay in 1971 for *Lancet*, Britain's leading medical journal, in which he applied Isaac Newton's inverse square law (for gravitational attraction) to medical care. He argued that those who needed care most were least likely to receive it. In gravitational terms, the farther someone was from the comfortable classes, or from a stable home and professional life, the weaker and less reliable the reach of modern medical treatment.

This bore special reference to the dying, who receive comfort and pain medications in proportion to their standard of living and the conventionality of their life. The poor, the culturally odd, the racially disfavored, the disfigured were more likely to spend their Last Days in warehouses for the dying, with inadequate pain relief; or alone at home; or on the street.

The point was outreach and a greater social conscience for medical institutions and the drug industry. The →Hospice Movement was one of the responses, as were free clinics and programs for low-cost cancer drugs, penicillin, insulin. There has been progress since 1971; but not enough. {→Politics}

What if we apply the inverse square law to the relationship between the Departing and those at the bedside? Is it true that the closer one is to the departure, the better the care--since there's always someone looking over the shoulder of doctors, nurses, orderlies. Obversely, is it true that the more remote the Departing is from you (emotionally, philosophically, physically), the less help s/he will get?

For some among the Departing, the Last Days are a rare and welcome time entirely to themselves after a life spent raising families, working in factories or offices, driving through traffic. The distance they keep at the end is a distance they embrace, its silence warm and restorative, bringing a person back to herself, or reconnecting with himself: a time for re-collection. {→Accidentals; Apples and Oranges.}

If you are at the bedside of such a person, do not take the silence as a repudiation of what you mean to the Departing. You are not being snubbed. Something else is going on here, which is not about you. You can help by assuring the quiet and privacy of the Departing, who do not mean to be leaving you in the lurch, and who will often come back for some moments before departure. In the meantime they need time to remember who they were, and are. The inverse care law turns out, at last, to be circular.

INVESTMENTS, DIVESTMENTS {→Money}

Capital gains tax on the sale of real estate or stocks by a surviving spouse is calculated not on the basis of the initial purchase price but on the market value as of the date of death of the Departed. For holdings that are not likely to increase substantially in market value over the next several years, the period immediately after departure can be an excellent time in which to sell, since there will be little or no capital gains taxes to pay. This is particularly true for widow/ers who are beyond eighty and do not need to plan for a secure income for the next fifty years.

That's the end of financial advice in this chapter. More important are the retrograde motions of investment and divestment during the Last Days. As departure nears, the Departing tend to divest themselves of earthly attachments while those at the bedside tend to invest more heavily in the Departed. How could it be otherwise? At the bedside you come to care physically and emotionally for the Departing in unusually intense ways that are surely appreciated, but such full appreciation cannot imply a reciprocal commitment to stick by you. For the dying, death does not endear.

A lucid if disconcerting economy is at work here. It is simply contrary to most habits or ideas of compassion to divest oneself of the Departing in the same manner or to the same degree that the Departing divest themselves from attachments to the living and a world in flux. This is not to suggest that deep affection or love dwindles as bodies grow cooler; it is rather to suggest that a certain distancing is more necessary and more natural to the dying than to those at the bedside. Do not mistake such distancing for anger, disaffection, recrimination, or sheer misanthropy {→Anthropology; Grumps}.

You are not to blame if and when it happens, nor are you to blame the Departing. Blame the stars if you wish, for celestial bodies also appear to shift their positions in retrograde motion, as if the Earth had suddenly started spinning in the opposite direction.

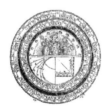

JERKINESS AND AGITATION

Muscle twitching in the arms, hands, and legs results either from the failing of the body's metabolism in the Last Months or as a side-effect of drugs. If drugs are the cause, the twitching can be stilled by lowering dosages or switching drugs, but the twitching may be more bothersome to those at the bedside than to the Departing, because no one likes to bear witness to motions that are iconic of agitation, seizure, or dementia. The use of tranquilizers or anticonvulsants to calm the twitching may therefore be mostly for the benefit of caregivers, unless . the Departing want to continue to feed themselves.

If accompanied by physical restlessness, flailing, tossing off sheets, and attempts to get out of bed, twitching may be a →sign of otherwise inexpressible pain, constipation, difficulty breathing, or high blood calcium levels. These possibilities should be investigated only after considering that the restlessness may be no more, **and no less**, than a final struggle to assert one's independence and mobility after weeks of inward fuming at an increasing dependence and immobility.

Emotional and mental restlessness may also manifest itself in muscle twitching as well as muttering or sporadic groaning, uneven breathing, spitting, or fear of being touched. Hospice nurses usually prescribe benzodiazepines for this; their favorite drug in this family is lorazepam (Ativan, Temesta), because it can be administered as a liquid under the tongue and works swiftly against anxiety, flashes of anger, and paranoia, all of which can interfere with the daily care of the Departing. In some people, Lorazepam has side effects serious enough to outweigh its benefits: terrifying hallucinations, heavy sedation or, oppositely, insomnia. Another family of calming drugs, serotonin 1A agonists such as buspirone (Buspar), are less likely to cause hallucinations or sedation, but they do not work as quickly. An alternative would be herbal preparations such as kava kava or marijuana. (The evidence for the anxiolytic effectiveness of St. John's wort is insufficient, and it has significant downsides.)

Keep in mind that, like yawning or coughing, expressions of anxiety and restlessness can be infectious. The more anxious or restless the Departing, the more you may begin to feel anxious or restless. You may then respond to the situation so vehemently or anxiously that you make the Departing more anxious: a jerky circularity devoutly undesirable.

JOKES

Gallows humor has a venerable tradition, and the Departing themselves may tell the bleakest of jokes, make puns in the worst taste. The Last Days need not be Days Aghast.

Indeed, with our late-evening talk shows hosted by comedians who do long monologues at the top of each show, our joking tradition is as much a custom of the night as it was in pre-modern times, where the voice still held forth by the embers of a fire. Lateness, darkness, jokes about death: exactly.

Many a cartoon depicts the Departed standing before pearly gates, or on clouds in Heaven, or on the way to Hell; far fewer deal with people at the bedside. An exception is a collection of cartoons edited by Mort Gerberg: *Last →Laughs: Cartoons about →Aging, Retirement . . . and the Great Beyond.*

Jokes, on the other hand, seem to move more easily between dying and death. For example, these are in the public domain:

A few days after Beethoven was buried, a couple strolling through the cemetery heard strange noises coming from his grave. Terrified, they ran and got the keeper to come and listen to it. He bent close to the grave and heard some faint, unrecognizable music. Frightened, he ran and got the town magistrate. When the magistrate arrived, he bent his ear to the grave, listened for a moment, and said, "Ah, yes, that's Beethoven's Ninth Symphony, being played backwards." He listened a while longer: "There's the Eighth Symphony, and it's backwards, too. Most puzzling." So he kept listening, "There's the Seventh. . . the Sixth . . ." Then he realized what was happening. He stood up and announced to the crowd that had gathered: "Fellow citizens, there's nothing to worry about. It's just Beethoven decomposing."

Supposedly true Inscription: On the grave of Ezekial Aikle in East Dalhousie Cemetery, Nova Scotia: "Here lies Ezekial Aikle, Age 102. The Good Die Young."

The method to most jokes is reversal of expectations through odd but logical substitutions, a switching of context. Why would the Departing not want to play with such transformative visions? Why should you not want to play along?

KEEPSAKES

Holdfasts would be the older, better word. As in, holding fast to a person. During Long Days and the Last Days, if at home and at the bedside, your eyes will light upon objects in the room that define the Departing: a painting that's been hanging in the same place for years, a bowl laid out just so, a scarf you remember from many a Thanksgiving, a well-worn book on a shelf, a pendant that's gone through hell and high water.

And when you think, as you will, that it would be good if you could have that bowl or book once the Departing has gone, the holdfast comes to mean "holding fast to the memory of a person," which is also a holding fast to the warmth of the person who cherished that object.

And when you begin to think seriously of what you would ask of the Departing --what one thing you would like to be given-- then the holdfast comes to mean "holding fast so as to keep one's footing": for such a gift is a tender of mutuality.

In some families, months before departure, the Departing label each likely keepsake by name, to avoid challenges in the Days After as to who gets the amber necklace crafted by a great-grandmother, who the pearl cufflinks salvaged after the fire. These are keepsakes because they have "sentimental value," a disturbing phrase that demeans the objects closest to us throughout our lives--"only sentimental value," after all, not a collector's item, not a major investment, so not mentioned in the →will. What can be sold for good →money is usually listed in a will; keepsakes often are not; holdfasts rarely.

The essential difference between keepsakes and holdfasts is the difference between memorabilia and touchstones. With memorabilia, one can reconstitute a person apart from the world and its density of relationships. With touchstones, at every touch the Departed returns to be held with you as part of a personally historic moment, a particular engagement of the mind, senses, heart.

During the Last Days, the Departing may also hold onto something. . . a linen handkerchief, a small clay figurine shaped and glazed by a child, a quarter (you would be surprised how many want the assurance of being able to give a tip). This keeps them in the world, despite the clearing out of the room to accommodate a hospital bed or medical appliances. It is not unthinking, this sort of holding fast. It reminds them of who they are, where they have been.

None of us wants to leave this life empty-handed.

KEYS

Metallic or musical? Both.

Security, privacy, and serenity--architectural *and* acoustic -- must be considered when at the bedside. {Also→Gatekeeping.}

Early on, everyone at the bedside must decide on a procedure for keys: which doors should be open, which locked, and when? Who should have keys, and who not? Who will be responsible for keeping track of the keys? (For example, if a paid caregiver is given a key but then quits, or an out-of-town relative goes home, who makes sure that house keys are returned?)

What sorts of keys do I mean? Keys to front and back doors, to the car or garage, to a home safe or weapons lockbox. There may also be keys for RVs, storage units, rental properties.

That's a lot of keys. If they are all on one keychain and held by someone with a nervous habit of jangling them, they will make a loud, dissonant sound that only an infant interprets as music. Keep hands off the keys until they are needed. (That goes as well for people of all ages who like to play chopsticks on the piano wherever it is and wherever they are.)

But back to the openings and closings. Assign one person or couple to keep track of all keys. Make copies of important keys and put them in a secure, memorable place in *another* home. Each person leaving the bedside should check that the proper doors are open/locked.

For a person at home who is seriously ill but alone for part of the day, whether for ten minutes or two hours, either the front door should be unlocked (for emergency access) or a close neighbor with a key should be on call, with a sign to that effect on the front door, along with a phone number and address.

Which brings me to paranoia. People in weakened conditions feel justifiably vulnerable and may be more fearful of strangers than ever before. Some →medications may cause paranoia or exaggerate existing fears. Stroke often animates deep-seated phobias or prejudices. Senility may be marked by a mounting fear of thieves at home or a conviction (in hospital or SNF) that there are plots afoot to keep a person awake or dehydrated.

So keys play a doubly significant role in assurances of security. It is vital that the policy of open/locked doors is fully understood by everyone at the bedside, and the location of keys is confidently known by all who should know. Otherwise, the bed and the bedside at home will begin to feel like dubious, if not dangerous, places.

LAST BREATHS

Romain Gary's *The Gasp* begins with a scientist capturing and preserving the final exhalation of a dying person. In that breath, *le souffle*, is the life-force, understood to be so powerful that an international philosophical thriller ensues.

Some people desperately want to be present at the moment of departure, as if the Last Days come to fruition in *le souffle*. Some are ambivalent, afraid of what they may find in that moment. Some would rather not be in the room at all; they prefer to remember the Departing in an earlier stage of farewell.

There are no attendance requirements during the →Last Hours. I have read thousands of →wills from all centuries and classes of decedents; not once have I come upon a bequest that is conditional on bearing witness to the Last Breath.

Nor is there any assurance that the second you slip out to use the bathroom or get the mail, the Departing will not, as it is said, *expire*. You can't ask the Departing to hold on.

Nor is there any assurance that you will be aware of the instant that the Last Breath has been let out. If the Departing has been →aspirating and has a rattle, you may notice in half a minute or so that a new quietness has fallen upon the room; if the Departing has been in a drugged sleep, you may notice after a longer while that the room seems a little too motionless; if the Departing has been talking and then, as so often before, has drifted off into silence, you may notice nothing for quite some time. In film and fiction, Last Breaths are more dramatic.

As a novelist, Romain Gary plays with the notion that the last breath has to be as special as the first, that passing on must pass on *something*, cannot be merely a passing out. "Passing out" is fainting; "passing on" sounds like dying *and* bequeathing, so it has to be dramatic, doesn't it?

If you are there for the last breath, and you hear it when it happens, what do you find? Quietness. Stillness. That's it. Almost never do you see a sudden trickle of blood from the mouth, a sudden clenching of fists or unclenching of features.

If you are not in the room for the Last Breath, what do you miss? A subtle moment of new quietness, new stillness. Rarely is there a deathbed confession with the Last Breath, or an *oh my*! or an *aha*! Those, if they come, come well before.

The sound that humans naturally make as they breathe out, a long last breath, is something like *Om* or *Amen*. *Om* with an *oh*. *Amen* with an *ah*.

LAST DAYS

Last Days imply a life beforehand, and a duration near the end. These pages can be of little help, sadly, to those faced with the passing of newborns, infants, young children. I had been, for as long as I knew, the oldest child in my family, but it turns out that I am the oldest *surviving* child. Before I was born, my parents had a child who died in the first week of life; they knew, from signs before birth, that the child would not live. There are books and websites that deal with such situations; this book does not {→Further Reading; Useful Websites}.

Nor will a book on Long Days and Last Days be of much help for those confronted with death at a distance, or on a battlefield. These pages are far less about →grief than they are about company, compassion, final conversations, and final embraces.

This book can be of limited help to those coping with departures via dementia, but when a person is unaware of time or place, it is difficult to be present *to* that person during Long Days or Last Days; one can only be present *for* the person. Neither neuro-physiologists nor physicians know much about →consciousness during coma, →delirium, or the later stages of dementia. {→Ageing,}

On the other hand, with advances in emergency and geriatric medicine, and with the global population of those over the age of sixty expected to double in the next forty years, Long Days and Last Days are going to be an increasingly common and shared experience. Already there are worldwide epidemics of lung cancer and HIV/AIDS in which patients linger, in need of all the wisdom and care we can muster. With global climate changes, Long Days and Last Days due to famine, drought, flooding, and contaminated water will arise not only in the poorest of countries but in regions once considered fortunate.

Worldwide there are some 100,000,000 persons who would benefit now from palliative care and →hospice groups. Access to such care is limited by poverty and lack of education, by ethnic rivalry or racial discrimination, by social or geographic isolation. Many would argue that freedom from →pain and abuse during one's Last Months and Last Days should be as much a right as a life lived free of hunger, in security and dignity. One cannot "die with dignity" entirely on one's own; dying with dignity requires a communal investment. This guide concerns community.

LAST HOURS

Whereas----. . .why am I starting this chapter with such a word? Are the Last Hours the preamble to a declaration, a new provision in the law?. . .

Whereas the Long Days may move imperceptibly into the →Last Months and the Last Months move almost imperceptibly into the Last Days, the Last Hours seem somehow clearer. At first they will be clear to veteran caregivers, to →ICU and →hospice nurses and physicians, then they will be clear to you, too.

Sleep will be appear to be deeper, and Cheyne-Stokes breathing somehow less noisy, which may simply mean that you have grown accustomed to it. As you have, also, to a face whose muscles are at rest, eyes inward or unfocused when open. So little fluids have been taken in that the drool of previous days has vanished, and the skin is dry, becoming cool.

It is also quieter, if you are in hospital, because most of the monitors have been unhooked. If not, they should be. {→Noise.}

You can sense where I am heading with this, toward a calm, well-anticipated departure. But. . . .

Whereas many deaths do involve Long Days and Last Months and a truly extended departure, some deaths are much more →sudden. With these, the Last Hours are a massive, wrenching condensation of Last Months, Last Weeks, Last Days, and you will not be prepared. Cannot possibly be prepared. Deaths from automobile accidents, tornadoes, drive-by shootings, unsuspected blood clots and associated strokes may not grant you a bedside. Death may occur before paramedics arrive, or in the corridor of an Emergency Room, or on the way to surgery.

A departure so abrupt is brutal; it's like shellshock and entails among family and friends a form of what we now call Post-Traumatic Stress Disorder. You will need →help in ways that caregivers who have been at the bedside usually do not. Going off by yourself will be a strong inclination: why keep your hand in a world so flat-out cruel? What's there to say about something so irrational, absolute, and uncompromising?

Eventually there will be something to say, and you will find yourself saying it, to someone. I don't know what that is, or who that will be.

LAST MEALS {also →Food}

Appetite diminishes as the departure nears. During the Last Months, people enter from all sides with homemade casseroles, muffins, herbal teas, soups, each with its restorative virtues. These may help maintain electrolytes as well as drinks like Gatorade; they may provide as much energy as Ensure.

During the Last Days, when there is difficulty swallowing (dysphagia), food is rather an offering than a meal. People bring food because it seems useful and personal--useful, really, for those at the bedside, who neglect to eat. Personal, in that they recall a mutual fondness for a certain dish.

Yet, since nutrition is as much a set of cultural premises about the inner body and outward figure as a science of metabolism and in/digestion, competing food advisories keep coming in from all sides, up to the end. I have seen a woman in her Last Hours offered a Whopper by one friend, tofu salad by another.

With ostomy →tubes or IV (parenteral) nutrition, there are proscribed and prescribed nutrients. Ostomy tubes can be blocked up by nuts, seeds, soda pop, mushrooms. →Dialysis patients also have strict diets, which may be mildly relaxed.

For those Departing who can eat and want to eat, most rules are out the window. They will eat small amounts, but eating now is more about mouthfeel than appetite or nutrition. An inch of a hot cinnamon roll, perhaps, or a sip of wine.

About the wine: at the end, off most meds, those who had been accustomed to daily wine or cocktails may have whatever they want. It is common, however, for the Departing to experience strong changes in taste preferences and new sensitivities to →odors. They may spurn their once-favorite foods or drinks.

So the legendary Last Meals of convicts on death row are hardly the same as the Last Meals of people about to die of "natural" causes, for whom it is "natural" to depart on an empty stomach. In the last analysis, Last Meals are for you who must be fully present for the Departing. Those who faint at the bedside due to dehydration or loss of electrolytes may briefly upstage the Departing, but this does not prove their devotion or deep love; they need counseling and sustenance.

The first time that the Departing stops eating and drinking, it is not definitively the end. There are likely to be several rounds of fasting and feasting, several Last Meals before the body says Enough! and the kidneys shut down and the mouth opens only for tastes of air.

LAST MONTHS

Obvious or subtle, when Last Months become →Last Days, longterm caregivers may breathe a sigh of relief while (other) family and friends spring into action. You don't want to hurry a person toward departure, or at least you don't want to look as if that's what you're doing, regardless of emotional, physical, or financial exhaustion. To celebrate the shift from Last Months into Last Days seems cold or grasping: at last I can get my share of the inheritance; at last I can live my own life.

When Last Days reverse and become Last Months, everything else also reverses. That guilty sigh of relief at departure can become, more often than any will admit, anger and guilt, both suppressed while celebrating remission. But the anger and guilt remain--anger that you will probably have to go through the same motions and emotions again, in a near-future, just when you had gotten a grip on grief, and guilt that you're not as happy about the respite as you say. How long can you be expected to maintain your own equilibrium in the face of such ever-imminent loss? Grief suspended is still more grief than joy, and more draining because more difficult to express.

When Last Months become Last Days, you tend to focus less on the body than on the essence of the person. When Last Days reverse toward Last Months, you tend to refocus upon the body and its amazing capacity for renewal, although you talk mostly about the resilience of the person: a beautiful white lie. Yes, people *do* make extraordinary recoveries, apparently by force of will or prayer or love; and yes, it is good that there will be more time now for penetrating conversations and visits across →generations. And yet . . . and yet, why can't some people recognize when it's time for them to go? Why do they insist upon living on, exhausting the patience, →money, and stamina of family and friends? Aren't these returns to life the acts of stubborn, selfish, clinging people? Only egoists or narcissists would blithely rise from the dead like this, unaware of how much they inflict upon the survivors, who have already stomached as much as was in them to stomach.

It's as if there's a race between you and the Departing, a race toward acceptance of death. Sometimes the Departing wins that race, which outsiders call wisdom or peace or grace; sometimes you win, and there are no good words for such a victory, only recriminations. But it's common for dying, like living, to proceed with uneven rhythms, heart-stopping pauses, odd astonishing leaps and glides, pratfalls and →cascades. They don't call it the Dance of Death for nothing.

LAST THINGS, OR THE ESCHATON

No matter how graceful the departure, during the Last Days at the bedside you're going to have moments in which you realize that this is your last chance to
...ask the Departing something you've always wanted to know;
...tell the Departing something you've always wanted to say;
...do something for the Departing you always meant to do;
...deal with issues between the Departing and someone else.

It will also occur to you to wonder whether it is your obligation to initiate conversations with the Departing on
...the nature of life and death?
...the possibility of an afterlife or plausibility of reincarnation?
...the reality of heaven/hell?
...the cycles of the cosmos and the paradoxes of eternity.

That depends.

Has the Departing expressed an abiding interest in those Last Things?
If no, then no, do not initiate such a conversation.

Are you hoping for a preview now that the Departing is so close to the Other Side?
If yes, then no.

Do you believe it's your duty to speak to these issues, whatever the Departing thinks?
If yes, then no.

Are you anxious about these issues and in need of consolation?
If yes, then no.

On the other hand, if the Departing has always been interested in these questions, or without prompting has begun to address these questions, then yes, by all means explore the Last Things. (Seriously, by *all* means: drawings, films, music, poetry, painting.) Even for the entirely secular, questions about the meaning of life and death acquire a new intensity during the Last Months. It is not up to those at the bedside to resolve the questions or to sort them out {→Framing}as would a classical philosopher, but it behooves all at the bedside to address the questions with a seriousness that honors the concerns of the Departing. {See also →Accidentals; Anthropology; Reflection.}

In sum: it is a breach of faith during the Last Days to recast dying and death for the Departing, as if the Last Things were in your grasp alone.

LAST WORDS

Spurious, garbled, or banal, Last Words rarely meet our expectations. Invested as they are with greater significance than first words (which seem haphazard or overdetermined), Last Words need to be at once capstone and inspiration, a pithy summation of a life well-pondered and a hearty admonition or encouragement to those who will be living on. Some sort of secret would also be good, an incident never before revealed.

The scenario is this: the Departing, just before →Last Breaths, looks around at the assembled company, gives a meaningful look in some direction, says something intentional, looks heavenward, and departs with a brief cough a few moments later. That "few moments later" is crucial. How else will the assembled be confident that those were the Last Words?

Imagine a novel put in motion by a controversy over one man's dying words. Was he exhausted, and did he say, "Let's call it a day"? Or was he still considering his options, and did he say, "Let's call in O'Dea"? Or was he waiting for a message, and did he say, "Les'll call any day"? And so forth. With every possibility comes a new context for the departure. There is such a novel: *Memento Mori* by Muriel Spark.

Last Words may not come at all. They may be overlooked because they come too soon. They may be half-heard because too quiet or too ordinary. They may be ignored as incoherent-- a cry of pain, a guggle. It is dangerous to look for all of a life, or a death, to be encapsulated in a single moment or phrase. Dangerous because, until the very end, we are minds and bodies in motion, not a succession of freeze-frames. Which means that there must always be some blur, some edge unfinished, some figure crossing suddenly behind us. To impose a strict and literate order is to insist upon death-in-life. Dangerous, also, because our lives are coherent only in the context of all the others who have stuck with us, not because of who we are but who we are with them. Dangerous, at last, because no words will suffice: they will be too few to do a person justice or too many not to worry over, pick at.

Last Words set us all up for disappointment or the misguided triumph of I-knew-it-all-along. Let it be as it is with first words, a remarkable but not prophetic event.

There is a Yiddish saying: you are born with a pre-determined but unknown number of words to →speak; when you reach that number, when you speak that last word, you die. Not a moment before. Not a sentence after.

LAUGHTER

Belly laughs come few and far between as one approaches the Last Weeks, not because laughter is out of place or insulting, but because it may be impossible for the Departing to laugh deeply without coughing, wheezing, or spitting up, or causing some monitor to go haywire, →tubing to go awry. That said, you should not refrain from making →jokes in good or bad taste, or from attempting puns subtle or stupid, simply because laughter (or fake grimaces) might ensue. Some quiet laughter, or the hint of a smile, may beam from the face in the bed, and that would be all to the good. {See also →Anxiety; Fear of Death; Grumps; Pain; Sadness.}

Laughter is a physiological and psychological conundrum, in that we cannot explain cognitively or neurologically how it arises, cannot account for its evolutionary value, have not assessed the consequences of laugh-deprivation. Where exactly is the funny bone? And why is it that we can't expect satisfactory laughter from someone who has to have a joke or a comic situation explained? Is the secret to laughter in the moment, in the sheer unexpectedness, or in the sense of an unexpected sharing?

Although we're even more in the dark concerning the origin of belly laughs and why sometimes we can't stop laughing (or giggling), we do know that such spasms of laughter are almost always in company. It's the society of laughter, its primitive sociality, rather than the nature of the pratfall or punch line, that seems crucial to deep laughter--the way that professional laughers in vaudeville used to get audiences to laugh at length with them just by laughing in front of them, on stage, aloud, at length.

It stands to unreason, then, that laughing together may be as deep a communion as you achieve during the Long Days and into the Last Days, you at the bedside, s/he in bed. If you are laughing with a visitor or another caregiver within earshot, bring the Departing into that circle of laughter, for it is also a circle of care.

For that very unreason, sick humor may also work, though scatalogical jokes (toilet humor) may come too close for comfort. {→Shit Happens.}

Whatever you do at the bedside, do not force lugubriousness on anyone, and in the Last Weeks, you may want to revisit that ambiguous maxim, He who laughs last laughs best.

LAUNDRY

Why does so paltry a subject deserve a page to itself? Let me list the reasons--a short laundry list about laundry.

1. →Bedsores can arise from sheets improperly laundered so that detergent or bleach residues remain or from wrinkles implanted when sheets remain in the dryer too long after the cycle has ended.

2. Due to the sensitivity of their skin after days and weeks in bed, the seriously ill and the Departing may suffer from bed linens that are too rough (old and frayed, or shoddy, or highly embroidered) or untreated with softeners during the drying cycle.

3. The number of sheets, mattress pads, pillow cases, and →blankets that need to be laundered each day can mount up quickly where there is →vomiting, unprotected incontinence, bleeding, leakage from wounds/dressings, drooling, or persistent picking at linen {→Floccillation}.

4. The →odor from unwashed laundry can become increasingly unpleasant, especially to the Departing whose sense of smell may be heightened, and whose own body odors can become pungent due to biochemical changes in sweat.

5. Detergents and bleaches used in laundry (and the chemicals in some fabric softeners or toss-in dryer sheets) themselves can cause skin reactions among the bedridden, so laundry must be done carefully, free of perfumes or harsh cleansing agents.

6. The seriously ill and the Departing benefit psychologically and emotionally from changes of clothing and bed linens. In so far as their environment has become restricted to a room or two, clean clothing and new bed linens (especially coverlets) can be the most dramatic and personal of changes of scenery. They may prefer certain colors as well as textures; listen to them. Even in hospital or a →SNF, the bedridden and those at the bedside have a say about bed clothes and coverlets. You can bring in a favorite coverlet, colorful shawls or afghans.

At home, it is wonderful when members of the circle of care volunteer to collect, wash, and dry the laundry two or three times a week. This is an enormous contribution, though woefully absent from the annals of departure.

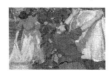

LAWYERS

Over hundreds of thousands of years, homo sapiens needed no lawyer in order to die. Indeed, as we learn from philosophers and poets, dying eludes the laws of humankind or unkind.

Nowadays only the dispossessed or defiant die without lawyers, who have drawn up →wills, →powers of attorney, trusts and, on the other side of the desk, terms for life insurance policies, inheritance taxes, and procedures for probate. {→Money.}

Those who do not own real estate or invent patentable products may never have professional contact with a lawyer unless it concerns the end of life. It's not death and taxes that are unavoidable; it's death and lawyers.

How common it is for those at the bedside to contemplate a malpractice suit. We are a litigious society, so the thought comes with a rush in times of inevitable nursing delay, technical mishap, drug reactions, medical miscalculation, or mishandling of the protocolsl for experimental treatments {→Iatrogenesis}.

Inevitable? Yes, inevitable. Physicians and surgeons may once have wished to be acknowledged as gods, and some may still hold themselves to inhuman standards of perfection, but they regularly make mistakes of judgment, practice, and personal relations, all of which are amplified by inhuman hours, crowded emergency rooms, and complex insurance regulations. Nurses, whose numbers in hospitals and nursing facilities are usually inadequate, make errors both of commission and omission, but also bear the brunt of complaints for problems originating in the contradictory, incomplete, or illegible orders of physicians.

I know of no one who has had impeccable care from Long Days through to the Last Breaths.

So there is always a handhold for lawyers and suits. The question is, a suit to what end? Justice? Aid for the next generation of sufferers? Remuneration for your travails?

Justice. Reformers often speak about justice. Outside of closing arguments, lawyers almost never do. And at the bedside, what does justice mean? Is it a euphemism for blood money? For comeuppance? Is it some sort of equilibration of pain: for so much anguish (yours? the Departing's?), so much shaking up of the medical establishment? Is it another name for the age-old attempt to establish an equation between laws of nature and human nature? Or is it a gesture toward the universe, a totem of defiant reversibility?

What would do justice to the Departed? And who?

LEMMINGS

Weighing in at 4 ounces, lemmings have done extraordinarily heavy lifting with regard to birth and death, all miscast. These furry, herbivorous rodents are not spontaneously generated from the northern air, as was thought in the sixteenth century, but they do breed in unusually chaotic cycles that, at the peak of an upswing, lead to large migrations. They are otherwise solitary creatures, indisposed to suicide, let alone mass suicide. The famous movie clips of lemmings following each other off a cliff into the ocean were fabricated for the Walt Disney Studio's 1958 Academy-Award-winning documentary, *White Wilderness.* A filmmaker in Alberta placed a few live lemmings on a snowy turntable and filmed them repeatedly until they became, by sleight of camera, a surge, which he then pushed off a short cliff into water below. [See Urban Legends, *Reference Pages,* 8 (1995-2005) by Barbara Mikkelson and David P. Mikkelson at www.snopes.com/disney/films/lemmings.asp]

At the bedside during the Last Days, you inevitably begin to think about your own death. Hypervigilant, you begin to notice in yourself symptoms of what must be an incurable illness {→Hypochondria}. This is similar to *couvade*, during which husbands take on the physical signs of a wife's pregnancy, including a swollen abdomen, dizziness, morning sickness. Anthropologists debate as to whether couvade is an act of empathy (I feel your discomfort), narcissism (look at ME, I am also with child), a ritual declaration of paternity (I share the pregnancy, since I am responsible for it), or yet another preemptive strike by patriarchy (man is the true childbearer).

Similarly, one can debate the significance of a sympathetic dying. Is it proof of your bond with the Departing? A cry for attention? A preemptive strike against the medical community (they can't heal the Departing, they're incompetent, not to mention unfeeling, so what can they do for me:→Iatrogenesis)?

It is true that some people lose the will to go on living once a loved one dies. You must tend to such people in the Last Days as earnestly as you tend to the Departing, watching for signs of despondent loneliness, abandonment of →medications, risky driving, long blanks in their →calendar for the coming months.

But there are also drama queens, cinematic lemmings, who claim that they cannot go on, that it is all too much, that the →Last Days are their finales.

Lemmings do not hibernate; active all year, they burrow in the snow to find food. In the wild they live for about two years.

LIGHT

Best to depart by natural light. I don't know why this is or whether statistics bear it out. (What statistics would I be looking for?) I don't even know whether a departure under fluorescent bulbs, halogen, or incandescence is somehow more problematic.

All I know is that natural light is best. And that you probably agree. During the Last Days, the Departing rarely gaze in rapture out the →windows or ask to sunbathe, and more people (yes, there's data on this) die at →night than during the day, so you needn't automatically agree with me. But I'll bet you do.

Originally I was planning to begin this chapter with an *aubade*, a song welcoming the sun in the quiet of the dawn. I would have composed a poetic sequence moving from dawn to dusk, with Dylanesque tropes about the dying of the light.

I thought better of it. I remembered the light coming through the living room windows behind my father's bed, and how the light suited him, how each day it differently suited him through to his departure one night near midnight. A lighting designer with all sorts of bulbs, filters, screens, shutters, and dimmers could have done almost as well, but it would not have been the same. Each second the sun turns 3,000,000 tons of hydrogen into pure energy, enough to light planets, moons, and clouds of asteroids billions of miles off, and yet when the sunlight streams through windows around the Departing during the Last Days, it falls gently enough to be just right.

Our atmosphere has something to do with this, and curtains, and angles of incidence. But one would have to be blind not to be startled then reassured by the rightness of the light. And by the rightness of the darkness in which the Departing so often choose to depart.

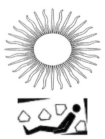

MEDICINE CABINETS

Economy and safety may be at odds here. All prescription drugs and most over-the-counter (OTC) medicaments are stamped with an expiration date; a formalist approach to safety would dictate that you discard any "expired" medication.

Most drugs, however, remain effective for years after the stamped date. As with the stamps on cans and packages of food, expiration or "best used by" dates are devised in part to assure manufacturers that retailers restock their shelves at profitable intervals. Drug companies are also being expedient about complying with a 1979 federal law that requires expiration dates on products but does not require proof of an accurate date for the potency of each drug. To be safe, they stamp a date that's almost always and extremely premature.

As explained by the Harvard Medical School Family Health Guide, citing research in *Pharmacology Today,* "Most of what is known about drug expiration dates comes from a study conducted by the Food and Drug Administration at the request of the military. With a large and expensive stockpile of drugs, the military faced tossing out and replacing its drugs every few years. What they found from the study is 90% of more than 100 drugs, both prescription and over the counter, were perfectly good to use even 15 years after the expiration date. . . . A rare exception to this may be tetracycline . . . . It's true the effectiveness of a drug may decrease over time, but much of the original potency still remains even a decade after the expiration date. Excluding nitroglycerin, insulin, and liquid antibiotics, most medications are as long lasting as the ones tested by the military. Placing a medication in a cool place, such as a refrigerator, will help a drug remain potent for many years." See the report at www.health.harvard.edu/fhg/updates/update1103a.shtml.

In a more recent (2012) study, California researchers tested eight common drugs that were in sealed bottles 28 to 40 years past their stamped expiration date. Of the fourteen active ingredients, including acetaminophen, amphetamine, aspirin, caffeine, codeine, and hydrocodone, all but amphetamine and aspirin retained a potency acceptable to the FDA (90% or higher). "All [the expiration date] means from the manufacturers' standpoint is that they're willing to guarantee the potency and efficacy for the drug for that long. . . . It has nothing to do with the actual shelf life," notes Lee Cantrell, a professor of clinical pharmacology and lead author of "Stability of Active Ingredients in Long Expired Prescription Medications," *Archives of Internal Medicine* 172 (26 Nov 2012) 1685-86.

This is important during the Long Days, when drug regimens change weekly and the numbers of prescription ointments, fluids, pills, and tablets mount up. It's also important because most of us have "expired" drugs in our medicine cabinets, and those cabinets are usually in bathrooms--the worst place to store pills and tablets, which deteriorate faster in warm, humid places. So, if the expiration date passed years ago, and if the half-used bottle has been sitting on a bathroom shelf, and if it's crucial for the pill to work at full strength, fill a new prescription. Otherwise, you may be able to rely on what's at hand. The government's own Shelf Life Extension Program allows drugs to be retained for 23 years after the expiration date if tests show that they remain potent.

The Johns Hopkins Health Alert advises, quite conservatively, "If your medications have been stored under good conditions, they should retain all or much of their potency for at least one to two years following their expiration date, even after the container is opened. But you should discard any pills that have become discolored, turned powdery, or smell strong; any liquids that appear cloudy or filmy; or any tubes of cream that are hardened or cracked."

Here are some specifics.

Storage: Unless refrigeration is specified, store medicines in cool, dry places out of direct sunlight, as in dresser drawers. Keep pills, tablets, capsules, and powders in their original bottles, but once opened (and before securely replacing the cap), remove any cotton packing that might wick moisture into the bottle. Antibiotics, ethyl nitrite and insulin must be kept in the refrigerator (above freezing and below 60 degrees F, so not in the freezer).

Preservation: Preparations that tend to dissolve, like zinc chloride, ephedrine, and digitalis preparations, must be kept in airtight containers with dehydrating agents. Ephedrine should also be kept out of the light, as should bismuth salts and quinine. Bacteria and fungi may grow in syrups, mucilage, plant and animal extracts, and in emulsions, creams, ointments, and injections. Chloral hydrate, calcium lactate, caffeine, codeine sulfate, and castor oil deteriorate quickly when exposed to air.

MEDICINE CABINETS, continued

<u>Asthma and other inhalers</u>: HFA propellants now used for inhalers are prone to absorb moisture once the inhaler is removed from its foil packaging, and moisture can cause the inhalant drug to clump, reducing the amount delivered at each puff. Better seals and the addition of ethanol to compounds have extended the effective life of opened inhalers to six months or more. Unopened inhalers appear to be good for three years after date of manufacture. No studies have shown any harm in using "expired" inhalers other than receiving less than full dosage from each puff.

Do Not Use:
melted or hardened suppositories, creams, medicated lotions, or ointments;
tetracycline that has turned brownish and viscous, regardless of expiration date;
expired nitroglycerin, insulin, procaine, arsenic preparations, and liquid antibiotics;
penicillin and cephalosporin when three years beyond date of manufacture, as also.
aspirin, amphetamines, hormones, vitamins, and liquid drugs over 3 years old.

For all unused **surplus** in your own medicine cabinets or that of someone who has died, →recycling programs through local pharmacies, state drug repositories, cancer associations, or international aid organizations are of little or no help. Most are legally obliged to discard all meds that have expired or whose seals have been broken, as must Drug Take-Back Networks. →After death, hospice nurses are instructed to sweep up all narcotics (and sometimes even all Rx) at home and destroy them, regardless of who wrote the prescription (e.g., a family doctor two years ago). In order to save non-hospice medications from such search-and-destroy missions, you may want to remove them from the home during the Last Days.

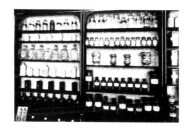

MEDICINES

→Caretaking at home, or at the bedside assisting a caregiver, you become responsible for the timely administration of medicines. During the Last Months, the Departing may be on a dozen or more drugs and ointments; typically the number will be reduced during the →Last Days. In order to keep track of complex medical regimens, it's best to work from two separate charts, as below. Since the charts will require frequent updating, electronic files are useful here. The first chart lists all medications (these are common in Last Days):

Medicine	Dosage	Start Date	On-Hand/ Refills	Purpose	Side-Effects	Notes
Roxanol =Morphine sulphate	Up to 1 ml= full dropper- p.r.n. but q4h	3/7	30 ml bottle =5-7 day supply	Acute pain relief	Constipation & drowsiness; if excess, paranoia	Put under tongue or inside cheek
Lactulose	1 tbsp q.i.d. Mix with fruit juice	2/24	473ml bottle =8-day supply	Relieve constipation	Diarrhea	Takes a day to work
Ativan =Lorazepam	1 dropper (=2 mg/ml) 30 min bef activity & q6h	3/7	120mg bottle = 2-3 week supply	Relieve anxiety, relax muscles	Grogginess; Temporary hostility or belligerence	Synergistic with morphine
Duragesic Fentanyl patch	100 mcg/hr 72-hr patch	2/20	2 boxes of 5 patches = 30 days	Relief of chronic pain	Dizziness; slowed breathing	No heat on or near patch

The second chart is for the daily round of medications. For example

Time of Day	Medicine	Dosage	Remarks
p.r.n. q4h	Roxanol	Up to 1 dropper	Use BEFORE pain sets in
p.r.n. q4h	Ativan	Up to 1 dropper	Use with Roxanol
1 hr bef breakfast	Levthyroxine	1 yellow tablet	Take with water
8 am / breakfast	Lactulose	1 tbsp	In fruit juice . . .
Through to 10pm	DuragesicPatch	Replace (every three days)	Put in new place on back each time
AND SO FORTH	FOR EACH	NEW	MEDICATION

Abbreviations:
~ approximately   < less than   > more than
s.i.d. once daily   b.i.d. twice daily   t.i.d. three times daily
q.i.d. four times daily   om once daily in morning
→ p.r.n. as needed
q4h every four hours   q6h every six hours
g gram mg. milligram   mcg. or ug microgram   kg kilogram
ml. milliliter (1 tsp~5 ml; 1 tbsp~15 ml.; 1 fluid oz~30 ml;
1 pint~500 ml.)

Note: While at the bedside you should inventory all medicines in the house (by location, name, dosage, expiration date, and purpose). You can review possible interactions at http://reference.medscape.com/drug-interactionchecker

MINDFULNESS

Many of these pages have been predicated on the assumption that you will be able to talk with the seriously ill and Departing, and that you will understand each other. Where Alzheimer's or other forms of senility are in advanced stages, or a person is afflicted by neurological disorders that have undone the →speech centers of the brain, or is in →pain so excruciating that the only charitable solution is an opiate sleep, there can be little or no conversation, and you must say your farewells without certainty that you have been heard {→Hearing}.

In these cases the Departing may sometimes wink, or wrinkle up a smile, or press your arm, or sigh. In degenerative diseases where the stages are understood, families and caregivers can work ahead of time with the Departing to arrange codes that substitute for each successive loss of a medium of communication: lip lifts, blinks, winks, eye motions.

So much of our sense of a person is invested in how he responds to a greeting, how she returns a gaze, that it is difficult to be mindful of a person who is silent and unresponsive. {→Anthropology; Identity; Laughter.}

For Buddhists and Taoists, mindfulness refers to a way of being that is alive to the world in all of its subtleties yet undisturbed by contradiction. A person with Amyotrophic Lateral Sclerosis (Lou Gehrig's Disease) may be alive to the world in many of its subtleties but appear to be utterly inattentive, as may also a person in late-stage Parkinson's Disease. To remain alive to the subtleties of someone who is Departing in silence, or in what appears to be gibberish, or with an obsessive paranoia, this is the most demanding of all efforts at mindfulness.

So, yes, I am taking mindfulness through all of its paces: the state of mind of the Departing; the neurological status of the Departing; our own state of mind with regard to a person who must depart without much of any farewell; and your capacity, at the bedside, to stay alert to the slightest signals.

None of us imagines for ourselves an involuntarily mute or disturbingly frightened departure. For that very reason, when you are at the bedside of those who cannot talk, cannot make sense, or cannot trust, there is a final mindfulness to be practiced: a recognition that the silence, the jabberwocky, the accusations are not directed at you, and that in so far as they have usurped the life of the person who is Departing, they should be paid no never mind.

Mindlessness. Mindfulness.

MONEY

Were you rich, there would be no Last Days, not now at least. You all could have flown to the best clinics and found what was wrong early on, before it was incurable. Money works wonders; those with less money experience fewer miracles. The rich need never worry about the grotesque cost of drugs or grueling appeals to insurance bureaucracies. They can hire the best live-in care. They may have access to new drugs not yet on the market, treatments available only in Europe or Asia.

While everyone is healthy, you may want to do something about these inequities {→Politics}. During the Long Days, you may draw up plans for later activism. But right now, nearing the end, there's no point in blaming capitalism or your own choice of a less-than-lucrative career. The rich die too, and in the Last Days their bodies go through the same decline. (In →hospice, many of the inequities are ironed out, though the rich may be able to pay for →agency →caregivers while the poorer must call upon →friends and relatives.)

Novels and films are full of people looking for money at the bedside of the rich. Devious or deadbeat distant relatives rush into mansions during the Last Days to be assured of a place in the →will, or to secure such a place, or to supplant others. Most people on the planet do not have much to bequeath.

Still, money gets in the way when thinking about paraphernalia for the hospital bed (fancy reading lights, unusually soft sheets) or about →funeral services and hardwood caskets. . . .You don't want to be stingy, and yet, wouldn't it be better to divert money from an elaborate memorial to improving the lot of the poor, diseased, orphaned? {→Plain Pine Boxes.} And is it sacrilege to think that all of the money invested in these last weeks could be put to better use funding pre-schools?

Some people, neither broke nor billionaires, have been paying life insurance premiums for decades. If money is a sharp anxiety during the Last Months and no policy beneficiary is impoverished, the terminally ill may opt to make a "viatical settlement," i.e., to receive immediate cash by reselling a policy to investors who now pay all premiums, gambling on the quick departure of the person covered by the policy, upon which they receive the full insurance payout.

At the last, the give and take of each enduring human relationship is not a market relationship. We do not bargain or barter our way into each other's hearts, and on departure no sales should be rung up.

MOTHERS AND FATHERS

Children are not supposed to die before their parents, but they do. In past centuries most parents had to cope with the death of at least one child. These days, infant mortality is much less, but a parent at eighty may still be called to the bedside of a son or daughter who is fifty or sixty. Even at sixty, the departure of that child can feel like a violation of the universal order.

Such grand language comes to the fore under exactly such circumstances. All cannot be right with the world when a (grand)father must bury a (grand)daughter, when a (grand)mother must choose the epitaph for a (grand)son. In consequence, mother and father may sacrifice their own health, and wealth, to save a child, moreso than a child would sacrifice to save a parent. Isn't this the way it should be? The universe replaces the old with the young, not vice versa.

>>Hard-hearted. Aren't children, who owe their lives to their parents, obliged to sacrifice themselves on their behalf?. . .To keep them alive for another five years?

<<You may wish to believe in full reciprocity. But the world cannot proceed on the basis of mutual self-sacrifice. The old must die.

>>Oh? At what age? Doesn't everyone have a right to die trying to reach the fabled 120 years?

<<No. The old should know when to leave. How many years of declining mobility, memory, and →eyesight should any body stand for? Why prolong the agony of a life without reach?

>>Honor Thy Parents.

<<But now you're the real parent, with powers of attorney, and your mother and father are the children. Now what?

>>You do everything they did for you, time and again, when you were ailing as a child. If you cannot return all the parental favors, you can at least assume responsibility.

<<For them as well as my own children? For how long?

>>Do you blame them for living as long as they have?

<<I blame them for not telling me everything I needed to know, so I have to be at the bedside waiting to hear the rest. I blame them for considering me a child long after I became an adult.
I blame them for accepting my apologies too readily, and for dying at the wrong time. Last month would have been better. Or next March.

MOTHS AND MINISTERING ANGELS

Certain individuals are drawn to the Departing as moths to candle flames. The simile is so exact it is impossible to avoid. Death Moths are warm people, soft of manner and quiet-spoken, who come around unsolicited to offer companionship with the Departing, whom they have met before in a casual sort of way. They are good night-time companions, for they do not ask much and do not mind silence or restless dreams.

In the long run, during →Last Months, their presence may become disconcerting, as they return each evening ever so gently insistent upon the momentum of their communion with the Departing, who has become as much their secret source as their center of compassion. Slowly but surely they can eat a hole in the fabric of family and friends as they tacitly lay claim to the inner life of the Departing, which through long nights or slow afternoons they have shared as if telepaths. They may become resident Fates to whom some look for guidance while others contest their monopoly of the bedside.

Death's-head Hawkmoths, so-called because of the skull pattern visible on the back of the thorax, are large moths, five inches long, of the genus *Acherontia*, species *atropos*, *styx*, and *lachesis*. In classical mythology, Styx is the river that circles the Underworld; Clotho, Lachesis, and Atropos are the Three Fates, daughters of Nox and Erebus (Night and Darkness). The insignia of Atropos, a veiled face above a pair of scissors ready to cut the thread of life, resemble a skull and crossed bones. Adult Death's-head moths raid beehives to suck out the honey, squeaking in imitation of the noise that a queen bee makes when it is about to lead a swarm. Make of this what you will.

Then there are Ministering Angels, people who have found that they have the gift of comforting those in their Last Days. Unlike →Bounty Hunters, Ministering Angels are truly focused upon the Departing and arrogate to themselves no special privileges by virtue of their powers. Because they have been at many a bedside, they may seem a bit too lighthearted, but they are practiced and practical and do not intrude themselves when the room is full or the Departing is dozing. {→Gatekeeping.} Where Death Moths cling and gravely flutter, Ministering Angels pass over, pass through.

A few may wish to, and need to, die alone. This solitude must be respected, and neither Moths nor Ministering Angels should then be admitted. Most of the Departing, however, welcome quiet company.

MUSIC

Mozart or madrigals or heavy metal? Strings or windchimes?
Bamboo flutes or baroque brass or drum machines and
screeching amps? Opera or light opera or musical comedy?
Rap or ska or scat or folk? Pop or rock or Gregorian chant?
Men's voices, or women's, or children's, or instrumental? Very
loud, sorta loud, soft, or way off in the background?

If music is personal, consider how much more personal it must
be once there are issues of →hearing loss due to age, acute
infection, or chronic illness, all with their accompanying drugs,
some of which over time are ototoxic and may do further
damage to the ears. Consider also issues of pain, anxiety, and
breathing problems that make one hypersensitive to certain
tones, timbres, and rhythms, oblivious to others. Then there is
the problem of ears-in-proximity: live-in caregivers, hospital or
→SNF →roommates with the tv going full-blast.

You may think to resolve this last problem by providing a CD or
MP3 player with earbuds, but you will need to evaluate manual
and digital dexterity, wrist strength, diminished vision, and
consider as well the prospect of terrible sensitivity around the
pinna of the ears. It's not easy to know beforehand who can
manage what device.

Thoughtful visitors often bring their own devices and a selection
of recordings that can be shared at the bedside according to the
whims and wishes of those abed. At home they may offer to
pull a particular record, tape, CD, or DVD off a shelf and play
that. Children may offer to play something on their own
instrument. . .this must be short. {→Young People.}

Whatever music is decided upon and whichever device is
started up, the seriously ill and Departing may have a spike of
energy and enthusiasm, or they may fall asleep after the first
strains, so deeply asleep that they snore. This is OK. You too
just might fall asleep. No one here is in a concert hall, and
music that "merely" relaxes may be just what the doctor
ordered.

Of course, the music might set the both of you thinking about
times past, or an old movie, or the resonant voice of a friend.
Do not shush a person who starts in talking above the music.
This is no music appreciation class, it's a bedside. Music may
be as close as you both come to a walking--a moving--
meditation.

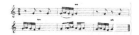

MUTUAL PERIL

Within the same week or month, wife and husband become seriously if differently ill. Or two sisters; or a mother and her caregiving son, a father and his caregiving daughter. They both need you at the bedside to make sense of test results, treatment plans, prognoses. They need you to plot the next steps, monitor medications, follow-up with doctors.

Of a sudden your own life is on hold. Worse, you cannot see a way to resume your own life in the near future. Everything here is too complicated, too foreboding, and you don't have the →money to hire a private →case manager to lift the burden.

Mutual peril is a phrase that redounds upon itself: the two who are frail or ill and can no longer rely upon one another for the foreseeable future; your life vis-à-vis the short- and long-term demands of the two; the well-being of those who rely upon you.

What do you do? You ask for →help: from →social workers; from →agencies public and private; from organizations devoted to a specific illness; from neighbors, friends, and relatives.

Why do you, competent, intelligent, and articulate as you are, need so much help? Because, often, one of the two will not admit that he cannot take care of the other, or that she cannot manage the household as before. Because one's issues are primarily cognitive, the other's primarily physical, and neither will be able to respond effectively to the condition of the other once back together at home where they insist on remaining. Because their rhythms of recuperation, and the extents of their recoveries, are rarely in sync. Because, perhaps, one is clearly now in the →Last Months, and the other is in no psychological shape to acknowledge or cope with the oncoming hardships.

So, yes, it's up to you to give them the respect they are due as a dyad that has been of mutual benefit for so many years. Make every effort to keep them together, but insist on daily help wherever they are, even at home, however intrusive they may believe that a third person would be.

If the dyad has been parasitic or mutually antagonistic (sticking together for years out of fear, habit, or a misplaced concern for reputation), then it's your obligation to separate them for their own healths, and for yours. This is hard. It involves painful discussions with family and friends, and you must be prepared afterwards to be accused of making the lives of the two sadder and lonelier in order to make your own life easier. Not so?

Not so.

NAILS

Everything else in disarray, fingernails and toenails continue to grow, catching on bedclothes, scratching at tender skin. Nails must be trimmed regularly--and carefully, so as not to cut into the surrounding skin. If a person cannot bend over, cannot see, or cannot handle clippers with precision, s/he will need help with nail care throughout.

For those who have thick, fungal, or ingrown toenails, it may be necessary to call in a podiatrist (yes, some make house calls).

Manicures can be performed by those at the bedside, so long as the Departing are not in the throes of →jerkiness or agitation; a slow manicure with warm water, lotion, and a deft touch can be equivalent to a massage.

People with autoimmune diseases (lupus, rheumatoid arthritis, HIV) and some cancers may develop vasculitis, one of whose signs is a series of small black spots around the fingernails. These cannot be erased by a manicure.

Because of the sensitivities of the Departing to →light and →odors and the likely presence of an →oxygen canister, never use acetone- or alcohol-based cleansers while performing a manicure. Fingernail polishes must be water-based; polish remover should be acetone-free and odorless.

Nothing is going to stop people who have been biting their nails for decades from biting their nails up to the end. Neither fear of God nor →fear of death has much effect on nail-biting. Do not interpret nail-biting as evidence of →anxiety, hunger, or melancholy. It is nail-biting, plain and simple, and there's really nothing for it. Who wants to be a nag now, anyway?

During the Last Hours, nails appear to turn blue: due to poor oxygenation, the skin beneath the translucent nails loses its pinkness. Do nails continue to grow after death? They appear to, as the skin around them dries and retracts, so that the nails look longer than before. In fact, they do not continue to grow.

As for your own nails, they should be short and smooth. This would seem to be a petty issue, but if you are helping change dressings or applying glycerin to the lips and lotion to the →hands and →feet, you will see the need for clipped, filed nails. With long nails not only is it difficult to maneuver among →tubes and apply gauze dressings; you risk scratching the Departing. You also risk making that horrible →noise called a "gride," like the sound of a nail scraping across a chalkboard.

Your nails will grow back.

NEEDLES

Needles: the very word may send some readers fleeing, so I come straight to the point: injections are slowly disappearing from Long Days and Last Days. In hospitals and skilled nursing facilities, injections are made mostly through IVs. At home the seriously ill may have implanted ports that accept special syringes that obviate the need to be stuck time and again in one arm or another.

A port is a small device usually placed just inside the upper chest or upper arm, where a →catheter is surgically connected to a vein. Inserted during an outpatient procedure that takes two to four hours from time of registration, it looks like a bump or lump on the skin. The port has a self-sealing silicon septum right under the skin through which drugs can be injected and blood drawn with little discomfort or chance of infection when properly prepped. A port can be used for months, although it may wear out and need to be replaced; unused for months, it may become unworkable or infected and need to be surgically removed in a shorter outpatient procedure.

Ports have different generic and trade names. Generic: totally implantable venous access system (TIVAS); central venous access device (CVA), central venous catheter (CVC). Trade names: Infuse-a-Port, Lifesite, Medi-Port, Microport, Passport, Port-a-Cath, PowerPort, SmartPort. Choice of port depends on its primary use: for chemotherapy infusions, blood disorder treatments, or . . . ? People with ports should carry on their person the name and version of their brand and the date the port was inserted.

In some situations, needles still loom. Hoping to ward off Deep Vein Thrombosis (DVT, blood clots) in patients bedridden while recuperating especially from strokes, hip or knee replacements, or stomach surgery, physicians in hospitals and →SNFs often prescribe daily Lovenox injections in the belly. These may continue at home if the patient is at enduring risk of blood clots. Lovenox (enoxaparin sodium) is an anticoagulant, technically a low molecular weight heparin solution (LMWH). It comes prepackaged as a filled-needle system easy to self-inject (see online video instructions). The needles are very thin, so the injections are relatively painless but there may be unsightly bruising, which can be mostly avoided if you don't rub or massage the area around the injection site.

NEEDLES , continued

Then there are needles for administering vaccines. Ordinarily, flu and pneumonia vaccines are given during the Long Days but not the Last Days. Live vaccines are usually contraindicated for those whose immune systems have been compromised by ongoing cancers, chemotherapy, AIDS, or antibiotic-resistant infections.

Two needles are used simultaneously with those kidney dialysis patients who have had fistulas surgically created in an arm or shoulder. Home dialysis patients can learn to operate the pair of needles themselves, or with help from others.

Finally, there are the needles--BIG needles--for cortisone shots for those with joint →pain, rheumatoid arthritis, or severe bone and muscle pain of unknown etiology. The shots themselves may be painful, but they work, sometime for weeks.

I mention these exceptions because Long Days and Last Months can be plagued by several distinct, possibly unrelated, problems. Steel yourself.

Oh, I forgot embroidery needles and knitting needles. Not long ago they were to be seen and heard around many a bedside, their quiet rhythms making for a visible and audible steadiness that could be genuinely comforting. I cannot guess how many coverlets, afghans, scarves, and sweaters must have been produced while →sitting at the bedside. but I don't see them very often any more. More disappearing needles.

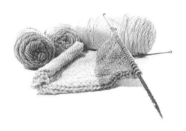

NIGHT AND DAY

Sunrise comes quietly at the bedside; sunset has a heavy presence. The placidity of men and women with dementia or Alzheimer's twists at twilight toward a disturbed →confusion and agitation. For those with macular degeneration, dimness itself makes the world more threatening, but otherwise it's our circadian rhythm of internal blood chemistries that's to blame for the "sundown syndrome."

Each of us has an autonomous bodily clock that runs closer to 25 hours than 24 with natural sleep cycles. Serotonin and melatonin, produced by the pineal gland, play a key role in keeping that clock regular and our mood swings minimal.

So night is internally distinct from day, and our internal periodicities in levels of enzymes, hormones, glucose, and circulating white blood cells may account for the greater frequency at night of heart attacks, asthma attacks, and strokes, as well as nocturnal flare-ups of ulcers, migraines, fibromyalgia, arthritis, and toothache.

The point is this: with night comes greater distress and →pain. For several reasons. At night, the pituitary gland, spinal cord, and brain produce less of their natural painkillers ("endogenous opiates") and perhaps less of the neurotransmitter dopamine, which dampens the intensity of pain. At night, people are more apt to panic at suspicious sounds. At night, insomnia due to breakthrough pain entails its own cycle of hypervigilance. At night, people feel their isolation more acutely: *Who do I call now? I don't want to wake my daughters, they've been looking haggard for days, and my doctor's not on call, I don't trust the others, and I really don't want a bunch of 911-firemen banging at the door and insisting on taking me to ER when all I need is →oxygen or someone to hold my hand, stupid, I should be doing the deep-breathing the nurse showed me, it's only 11:01 and I think I've already used up my pain pills--who cares if I get "overmedicated," totally zonked, all I want is to sleep anyway, but will I fall again trying to get out of bed why did they have to put the pills out of reach I should be in control here not them and make it through the night for once without bothering anyone I must be a royal pain but there it is it won't go away by itself, pain is pain, or is it all in the mind or those neuro-whats yes my thoughts are racing I'm supposed to slow them by laying my fingers on my inner wrist well and good in a doctor's office but with this splitting headache when did that start and it's not even 11:08 maybe I should call when it's 11:09 that's like 9/11 right?*

NOISE NOISE NOISE

Never will it be as quiet in a hospital or nursing facility as at →home, but being at home is no guarantee of quiet. How close is the bedroom to heavy honking traffic, bawling infants, peacocks, or a tv set boring through apartment walls?

That said, the central question is whether those abed are as concerned about noise as those at the bedside, who tend to be overly protective, keeping the environs safe from all intrusion but also secretly enjoying an unusual power that comes of being a sort of acoustic guardian.

Quiet can be recuperative. When recuperation is no longer the issue, some degree of noise may be welcome. That will depend.

In pain or anxious, the Departing become hypersensitive to sounds of all kinds. Hissing, screeching, or crashing noises can themselves be painful, and may exacerbate the pain of disease or injury. Hypersensitivity can make less abrasive sounds -- bumbling, shuffling, or busybody noises--equally upsetting. If you tend to wear long earrings or tinkling metal jewelry, you should watch to see whether the Departing winces as you shift in your seat or move around.

For those who are not in pain, a modicum of noise may be a delight, a sign of still being engaged with human affairs. To promote an unearthly stillness around the bedside can be frightening because premature and ghostly: an intimation of the crypt. For similar reasons, do not whisper in or just beyond the hearing of those abed; whispering near the bedside can only seem furtive, ominous

We are all fundamentally noisy beings, continually reminded of our bodies by burping, coughing, sneezing, snoring, snorting, belly rumbling, and farting. Our departures too may need some accompaniment, some evidence that we have been among the living and do not leave simply to find silence.

Some people will enjoy background →music, others will want nothing but brief periods of conversation or a silent sharing of the calls of birds beyond the →window sill. Take the hints.

During the Last Days, the Departing will likely be making some unusual noises due to periods of apnea or →aspiration, phlegm in the throat, or semi-hallucinatory mumbling. You in turn may become hypersensitive to sounds, trying to guess which of the Departing's noises are meaningful →signs of a change in status, and which are incidental. What should you listen for, a death rattle or the silence after?

NOMENCLATURE

English is clumsy at describing process, for which it relies heavily on participles: be*ing* born, dy*ing*. In the first days we have babes, babies, bairns, bambinos, bantings, buds, infants, little ones, neonates, nestlings, new additions, newborns, nurslings, one-day-olds, papooses, sprats, sucklings, tads, two-day-olds, three-day-olds, tykes, weanlings, and whelps, but for the process there are few words and phrases, often indefinite and awkward: bearing a child, birthing, giving birth, delivering, going into labor, having a baby, producing an heir and, technically, parturition. {→Mothers and Fathers.}

In the Last Days, the reverse holds true: few, and awkward, phrases for the dead--cadavers, corpses, the deceased, decedents, the defunct, the departed, the moribund, stiffs--and a more extensive, more colorful set of words for dying: biting the dust, breathing one's last, buying the farm, cashing out, checking out, croaking, crossing the bar, departing, down to the final count, enjoying one's last meal, expiring, fading away, fading out, failing, flat-lining, freeing the spirit, giving up the ghost, going home in a box, going to the happy hunting grounds, going to meet one's maker, going to the last roundup, handing in one's chips, heading out one last time, joining one's ancestors, kicking the bucket, leaving the building, letting go, losing one's life, making the supreme sacrifice, meeting one's end, passing away, passing on, passing over, perishing, pre-deceasing, relinquishing one's life, shuffling off this mortal coil, slipping one's cable, succumbing, and taking a turn for the worse, which is something of a euphemism, as is closing one's eyes, dropping off, going to →sleep.

Aside from "dying" and "the dead," the only pair of words common to both the process and conclusion are "departing," "departed." These are the words I have chosen for this book, because they allow, literally, for more departures, medical and meditative, practical and philosophical, emotional and relational. If these words seem less blunt, they are not euphemisms. The point of being at the bedside during the Long and Last Days is rather to accompany, and perhaps ease, a departure than to bear witness to a dying and a death. The media give us death and dying every hour, in daytime cartoons and soaps, in nightly news and police procedurals, in feature films and webcams. Departure is different: together, the Departing and those at the bedside share in the crafting of days that are neither generic nor tidy. "Departure," more than any other word in English, takes into account a time at once retrospective and prospective and, I would hazard, sufficiently open-ended.

NOT WANTING TO KNOW

Ethicists argue that the Departing have a right to know, and an equivalent right not to know. Not to know anything about the illness or its prognosis. Not to know how many weeks they may have left. Somewhere along in there, they probably do know, but they also have a right to pretend not to know.

Families may decide for themselves that the Departing should not know. This raises questions. Should the Departing be left in the dark so that they do not lose the will to fight (against cancer, multiple sclerosis, the complications of lupus)? Or because prognoses are often wrong--in one direction or the other? {→ETD}. Or because a cure may be just over the horizon, if only the family can scrape together the cash for a trip to a remote clinic? Or because they would become angry, hysterical, unmanageable, a greater burden than before?

It's unlikely that the Departing will not know when they have come to their Last Days. Possible, but very unlikely. Whether they indicate that they know, that's another matter. They may suspect that you don't want to know that they know, because you want them to fight on up to the very end. Or they may suspect that you will get hysterical and unmanageable once you know they know, and you will be of little help at the bedside.

Entering palliative care or →hospice, everyone knows that the end is nigh, but no one knows exactly when. →Counting down is a mid-20th-century habit that serves no good purpose during the Last Days. There is a substantial difference between having six months to live or a week; how much difference is there between forty hours and forty-three hours?

The right not to know can mean the right not to have diagnostic tests that would help establish a →calendar for the departure. This may be aggravating, this refusal to allow a calendar to be set, because it seems unfair to all who must break from their busy lives to be at the bedside. If the Departing do not need a calendar, the rest of us do, don't we?

Not wanting to know, then, is never a blithe choice. Consider for yourself: Would you like to know beforehand the date of your death? If so, how long beforehand? If not, how can you make reliable plans? And in either case, how will you live your life differently? What would change as you move through your Last Days?

NOTHING FUNNY ABOUT THIS

Classically, a comedy is a drama in which all ends well. Can a drama that ends with the death of the central character ever end well? Yes it can. With a →sudden death? No. With a mean or dispirited death? No. With a painful death? Possibly, for then death may be a welcome release for the Departing and a relief for those at the bedside. With an anticipated and completed death? Certainly.

A completed death is one which the departure has few loose ends, in which what had to be said has been said. A completed death is one in which there has been time enough for the Departing and those at the bedside to make their peace with each other and with the departure itself. A completed death is comic not because there have been pratfalls, doubletakes, mistaken identities, or groaning puns (all of which there may well have been), but because in the Last Hours and in the Days After people tend to smile, grateful to have had the time they did with the Departing, or grateful that the departure was neither physically nor emotionally punishing.

It is tempting to confuse the genre of comedy with utopian notions of "a good death" and "an easy death" {→Deaths, Bad and Good}. There is nothing utopian, however, about how this very human comedy plays out. Smiles at the end are hard-won and last only to our next travail.

The opposite of comedy is tragedy, not seriousness. In classic tragedy, the death of the central character arrives as a brutal reversal of fortunes or indiscriminate disaster (a fire, an accident, a car bomb) just as someone is about to achieve a dream. Comedy makes fun of shock; tragedy suffers from it.

Melodrama pretends to tragedy, but characters in a melodrama takes themselves too seriously, inflating everything into crisis. Everything is so fraught with serial repercussions and passions that no life can be lived with grace. Overmuch →sadness at the bedside tends toward melodrama, bad melodrama, where actors and actresses upstage each other and the Departing.

As comedians say, comedy is a serious business, because we →laugh hardest at that which is most meaningful to us and at that which changes how we think about our world {→Jokes} The Long Days and Last Days are therefore prone not only to black humor but to a belly-laugh here and there.

The word "funny" has its origins in the word "fond." Among →friends, then, there is something funny about departure, and one hopes it will be comic, as in: ending well.

NURSES, NURSING

LPNs, LVNs, NPs, MSNs, RNs . . . such an alphabet soup of nurses these days: Licensed Practical, Licensed Vocational, Nurse Practitioners, Masters of Science in Nursing, Registered Nurses). Many are specialists watching cardiac monitors or working exclusively in surgical ICU {→Intensive Care}. Some go wherever they're assigned. Because they are still "nurses" (recall the origins of that word), we expect all of them to be liberally gifted with TLC. Yet they often have too many patients under their C each shift--and precious few minutes for T, let alone L.

Unless you've hired a private LVN or a live-in CNA (Certified Nursing Assistant), it's up to you to watch for what may escape the harried glances of nurses.

As a nurse-substitute, what should you be watching for?
→bedsores.
--blood leaking from an IV tube (or →catheter) insertion site, which can indicate a problem with →tubing, veins, or tissue.
--difficulties swallowing, which may require a repositioning of head and throat and special thickened liquids {→Food}.
--difficulties breathing {but →Aspiration, Oxygen}.

When someone is on a complex regimen of drugs, you may also need to remind nurses at hospital shift changes or visiting RNs at home about →medications added or deleted, dosages raised or lowered. During the Last Weeks, you may also need to record the times and amounts of morphine dropper use or the finishing of a fentanyl sucker.

At the bedside hour after hour, you will be more adept than any nurses at judging the level of →pain of those who tend not to ask for relief until the pain has become unmanageable.

You'll wonder whether you are making a nuisance of yourself, and whether such assertiveness leads to worse care, because nurses tend to avoid a "difficult" room and delay responding to further outrageous requests. But so long as nurses are treated with respect, and not as servants or bellhops, you can be an effective →advocate. So long as you explain why you think that something strange or awful is going on, you will not be avoided, particularly if you can help the staff understand the desires or discomforts of the ill or Departing. Nurses in turn can help you understand what is odd and what is normal.

In none of this can you be shy. Nor can you shy away from the blunt language of sweat, blood, piss, →shit, diarrhea, drool. Even as the body demands less, more may be demanded of you.

OBITUARIES AND OBSEQUIES

Small local newspapers and a few metropolitan newspapers publish obituaries free of charge. You must write up the "death notice" to fit a specific format and length; longer texts, or texts with photos, incur a charge. Since newspaper deadlines run a week or more ahead of publication, you cannot always rely upon a print obituary to provide the community with timely details about a funeral or memorial service.

Obituaries can also be posted to the web quickly and reliably. For-profit memorial websites post obituaries for a fee that is frequently less than a newspaper's charge for a death notice, especially if you want to include a photograph: Click on Obituary Depot at www.daddezio.com/obituary/links.html

Obituaries are written, public notices of a death. *Obsequies* are →funeral ceremonies that include an invitation to mourners to speak about the Departed. *Eulogies* are more formal orations, usually composed beforehand and intended for publication afterward. Because eulogists customarily praise the Departed, the word has come to refer more loosely to any exaltation of a person retiring or "moving on," but it is most moving as a thoughtful summary of a life in its entirety, warts and all. An *elegy* is a poetic or musical eulogy; elegiac verse, music, or art blends the melancholic and insightful. A *wake* was once (<Old English *wacian*, "to be awake" and "to keep watch") a death watch at the bedside, then a watching over the body of the Departed in the hours before burial; today it is a festivity after interment, with food, song, and eulogies quiet or uproarious.

The Departing may want a say in their obituaries. Some may have drafted an obituary, or joked about doing it; others may appreciate a conversation about what belongs in their obituary. The tendency in short obituaries is toward a lifeless prose in which the merits of the Departed are listed as if on a ledger, along with some begats and flat statements of sorrow: "will be missed." Such language has traditionally been constrained by the column-inches of newspapers as well as the hurry in which obituaries are composed to meet deadlines. Working before-hand with the Departing on an obituary, a eulogy, even an elegy, you may elude these restraints.

Neither obituary nor eulogy nor elegy can be the final word. No person can be summed up in twenty-five words or ten minutes. Think rather of making sense of something about the Departed that always puzzled you, upset you, astonished you. And realize that brevity can lead to surprising, astonishing choices of what to say.

ODORS

Writing on "The Smell of Death," Abraham Verghese, M.D., describes "the mousy, ammoniacal odor of liver failure, an odor always linked to yellow eyes and a swollen belly; the urinelike odor of renal failure; the fetid odor of a lung abscess; the acetone-like odor of diabetic coma; the rotten-apple odor of gas gangrene; the freshly-baked-bread odor of typhoid fever. . . . the smell of unremittent fever in AIDS, fever that has gone on not for days or weeks, but for months. It is the scent of skin that has lost its luster and flakes at the touch, creating a dust storm in the ray of sunshine that straddles the bed. It is a scent of hair that has turned translucent, become sparse and no longer hides the scalp, of hair that is matted by sweat, and molded by a pillow."

One could write also of less telling but prevalent smells at bedsides, especially at institutional bedsides--flatulence, staleness, foot fungus, salt-seamed sweat.

Smell is our most unmediated sense. Neurophysiologically, our noses have a direct line to the brain, which is why odors are so tightly bound up with specific events or people. Those of the bedridden with multiple sclerosis, diabetes, Parkinson's, or Alzheimer's may have lost much of that pungency (a loss called hyposmia). Some will have distorted or hallucinatory identifications of smell (adysosmia or aphantosmia) due to alcoholism, nicotine addiction, or opiate overdose. In others, the perception of odor may be so heightened that they respond to the least whiff of putridity or aroma of blossom.

For those who are seriously ill, who have had their worlds circumscribed and their senses of vision, touch, and taste dulled by opiates, sedatives, and loss of saliva, smell may be almost as critical as→hearing, and perhaps sharper.

That the Departing develop an accentuated sense of smell is not yet supported by the medical literature; it is anecdotal and may arise from desires to promote aromatherapy or sell flowers or flower-scented air sprays and incense. It may arise from association with taste abnormalities that are common at the end. It may arise from the desire of those at the bedside to eliminate the remaining smells of death by projecting upon the Departing themselves an extreme sensitivity to smells. There is more to this, however, than sales(wo)manship or disguised disgust. There is something about being still, and still alive, that encourages a most subtle olfaction.

ORGAN DONATION

Kidneys, liver, heart, heart valves, pancreas, lungs, eyes, bone, tissue . . . the list grows year by year as to what can be "harvested" from the dead and even from those about to die. An ultimate altruism, you might say. Or a final abomination, a rude violation in those fateful minutes when souls are still floundering, not yet fully released from the teguments of flesh.

The Department of Health and Human Services tells us (at www.organdonor.gov) that one organ donor can save up to eight lives, and that 110,000 Americans are currently waiting for an organ. Blood type, tissue type, and body size determine recipients, so it is rare for a donor to be able to specify who gets what, which makes for an altruism blind to color, creed, ethnicity, political bent, or moral caliber.

I doubt that any physician decides to treat the terminally ill in a way that will best preserve their organs for donation. the Departing, however, may opt for one medical regime over another because they harbor a desire to be the best of donors. I would guess that this is rare, but who knows?.

Such gifting is territory for medical ethicists and for debate among co-religionists. Each religion does provide guidelines for, and more or less severe restrictions upon, organ donation. (Christian Science and Shintoism discourage them; Jehovah's Witnesses forbid them outright.)

Here I simply lay out the various technical options.
1. Donating one's body to a medical school for instruction.
2. Donating one's body for more generic medical research.
3. Arranging for an autopsy at a medical institution, apart from any autopsy by a coroner. (Private autopsies are pursued when the etiology of a fatal condition is mystifying or controversial, and/or when the family has an interest, genetic or otherwise, in resolving the matter.)
4. Designating one's body for organ and tissue donation.
5. Specifying in a will an intact burial or cremation.

In cases 1-3, retrieval of the body at death is usually effected by the designated institution rather than by a mortuary. In cases 4 and 5, "harvesting" is ordinarily done in hospital, with the remains given (as arranged) to a mortuary. Research institutions and medical schools have different policies as to what will be done after they have finished with the body: some will cremate; some will return the body/parts to a designated mortuary; some will not tell you what they will do.

OVERNIGHT BAGS (the minimum)

Clothing*
bedclothes
a change of socks/stockings and underwear
running shoes (if you go running in the morning, don't stop)
a windbreaker (for rain, for walking or running)
& check the weather (do you need a warm coat? hat? gloves?)
*If you expect an imminent Departure, pack more formal wear.

Toiletries and Devices
toothbrush, paste, and floss
nail clippers
hairbrush/comb, and perhaps a portable hair dryer
unperfumed soap or bath gel
neutral deodorant (no strong perfume)
hypo-allergenic lotions and cosmetics

Medicines etc.
your own prescription drugs** and supplements
something for a cough (coughing at the bedside is a real pain
for everyone)
something for constipation (after sitting a long time . . .)
vitamins (esp. C and E for resistance to institutional infections)
over-the-counter or prescription eye drops
prescription eyeglasses, sunglasses
**pack more of each than you think you'll need--if a visit lasts
longer than you expect, the only things that you won't be able
to borrow in a pinch will be your meds and prescription glasses.
Getting a new Rx is a hassle.

Wallet/Purse Items
driver's license
ATM card / credit card
cash in 1s, 5s, 10s (nothing larger than 20s)
8 quarters (vending machines, parking meters)
your own medical insurance cards
AAA card or other for hotel/motel discounts
address book: doctors, hospitals, emergency contacts

Additional
rechargers for cell phone/laptop/tablet
a pocket notebook and two pens
fine-tipped marker (for labeling items at the bedside)
duct tape or Gorilla tape (you never know...)
digital recorder or smartphone for recording conversations
{→History, Part I and Part II}
pillow or neck rest for long airplane trips

And, of course, your passport if crossing a border.

OXYGEN AND AIR

Once the breathing of the Departing becomes labored and secretions accumulate in the back of the throat, oxygen is introduced through small green tubes that fit into the nose. This is such a common sight that soap operas are incomplete without one such scene weekly, although designers choose more visually intimidating transparent masks that cover mouth and nose. The tubes, which look flimsy and may irritate the nostrils, are less dramatic than a mask but no less effective.

In →SNFs or at home, the oxygen comes from an unsightly canister whose pump can make a hissing or swooshing sound. There may also be a CPAP (continuous positive air pressure) machine at work, to ensure even flow for those with serious lung problems or →sleep apnea. Some people are so disturbed by the related →noises that they choose to do without.

Question: Why give those at death's doorstep extra oxygen? *Answer*: Even for the calmest, a basic fear of being smothered or strangled may cause intense panic when straining to breathe. Low levels of oxygenation (hypoxia) can cause hallucinations or exhausting tremors. Improved oxygen flow helps maintain an audible voice and mental clarity.

Still, that canister is an awful presence, and it makes its own emotional atmosphere. There must be no open flame in the room (e.g., matches, candles, cigarette lighters, incense), even when the oxygen is turned off. Nor must there be any fumes from rubbing alcohol or alcohol-based towelettes, mouthwash, deodorants. Canisters may have infinitesimal leaks, and pure oxygen is very explosive.

An oxygen canister in the room may lead caregivers to consider air filters and ionizers. Avoid these. Although high-tech "clean rooms" and hospital isolation units have their air scrubbed, all domestic air-cleaning machines are much too weak to make a difference in any room larger than a closet. Ionizing machines can release dangerously high levels of ozone. If the seriously ill or Departing insist, obtain a High-Efficiency Particulate Air (HEPA) or Ultra-Low Penetration Air (ULPA) filter/purifier.

Patients are now instructed to take deep breaths every couple of hours, so as to improve oxygenation levels. (At home, fingertip oximeters can be used by visiting nurses to measure the amount of oxygen in arterial blood by slight changes in blood color.) If at the bedside you find yourself nodding off, you may be tempted to borrow the Departing's oxygen; instead, take deep breaths. Deep breaths.

PAIN I

Pain does not translate and is incommensurable. My pain is not your pain, and on a scale of 1 to 10, a pain level of 8 today is not the same as an 8 tomorrow.

I have watched nurses and doctors ask about pain levels and seen them become annoyed as patients struggle with a scale that is literally treacherous. If a person names a number too low, he is in jeopardy of going untreated. Name a number too consistently high, and she is in the double jeopardy of being mistrusted or being knocked out. Name a number that waffles in the middle, and there are the triple jeopardies of being misunderstood, overmedicated, or undermedicated.

And which pain are they asking about? The bone pain of metastatic cancer is fierce but dissimilar to the splitting headaches of migraine, which are unlike the shooting and sharp pains of neuropathy. →Cramping is like the pressure pain of bowel obstruction only not quite, and very different from the slicing/tearing pain of damaged tissue or the raw abrasive pain of deep bedsores, which can be confused with some nerve pains but not nearly identical to the joint pain of rheumatoid arthritis. . . Enough of this.

If a patient manages to sum up the various kinds of pain into a single number, that number is good for maybe ten minutes. Pain changes with body heat and room temperature, with →sadness and sharp words, with onslaughts of →noise from corridors or hospital →roommates roaring with their own pain. The greater one's pain, the more intimate it may be, and the more inexpressible.

Like referred pain, which exasperates because it operates out of focus. The "referral" is deceptive: pain that is felt far enough away from its origins as to seem independent is called referred pain not because →physicians know the origin but because they know that the pain is not directly related to what lies directly beneath. How deal with it except by suspecting the entire body of collusion in the torture: a physiological McCarthyism.

Before the Last Days, pain might mean something important, might be information that can be used to diagnose and treat, even when "referred." During the Last Days, it is useless to try to find meaning in pain. This is no fitness center; there is nothing to be gained from pain, little to be gained from trying to determine the source of the pain. What the Departing needs, and deserves, is freedom from pain, as much as possible for as long as possible. {See next chapter→Pain II}

PAIN II

No one drug or therapy can eliminate all kinds of pain.

Why not?

Throughout the body are nociceptors, nerve endings that specialize in sensing different kinds of pain. Some respond to pricking, squeezing, pinching, or knifing and produce a sharp, local reaction transmitted to the spinal cord through A-beta and A-delta nerve fibers. Some respond to thermal or chemical stimuli or internal pressure and produce a throbbing, diffuse pain transmitted more slowly by C fibers. And some pain is neuropathic, i.e., nerve endings themselves are injured and firing abnormally, leading to spasms of sharp pain, long episodes of throbbing pain, or both. {See also→Pain III}

From the spinal cord, pain sensations are sent to the brain: the thalamus, the cerebral cortex, the hypothalamus, and the brainstem.

The brain responds first by activating two neurotransmitters, serotonin and noradrenaline, that modulate the pain along "inhibitory neural pathways."

Most pain-killing drugs and procedures--opiates like morphine, fentanyl, and oxycodone, as well as less powerful derivatives, like codeine; non-steroidal analgesics like acetaminophen (Tylenol); opiate-acetaminophen compounds (Percocet, Vicodin); hypnosis; deep relaxation--work at the level of the cerebral cortex and spinal cord, where they bind to opiate receptors or act upon them to release the body's own analgesics: endorphins and enkephalins.

Steroids, like cortisone or prednisone, and non-steroidal anti-inflammatory drugs (NSAIDS) like aspirin, celecoxib [Celebrex], ibuprofen [Advil, Motrin], and naproxen [Aleve]) work on the A and C nerve endings as well as at the level of the dorsal horn of the spinal cord.

Local anesthetics, like lidocaine or bupivicaine, block A and C fibers from sending pain signals. Cannabinoids (marijuana) also slow the transmission of nociceptor signals.

Acupuncture seems to work at many levels, from the A fibers to the spinal cord and the cerebral cortex.

Now you may understand why different painkillers may be used simultaneously. Opiates help with skin and deep tissue pain, often with abdominal and thoracic (or visceral) pain. Radiation and NSAIDs help deal with bone pain, which can be extreme. Neuropathic pain is often the most difficult to treat; opiates are usually of no help, and the most commonly prescribed drugs-- gabapentin (Neurontin) and pregabalin (Lyrica)--work by routes we do not grasp, so their effectiveness is hard to predict.

Some also try TENS, transcutaneous nerve stimulation to affect A fibers. Anti-anxiety drugs such as lorazepam (Ativan) and diazepam (Valium) may reduce all kinds of pain by reducing the stress. Hypnosis, light massage, and aromatherapy may also relieve anxiety and reduce the cognitive perception (if not nociception) of chronic pain, as may anti-depressants. Recent research shows that fully immersive environments (meditation, biofeedback, virtual reality goggles+headsets) may protect against chronic pain better than morphine.

What should you make of such detail? What's the "take-away"?

It's this: **Do not wait until a person is screaming or groaning or thrashing to administer pain relief**.

Chronic pain is much more than acute pain that has not gone away. The longer that pain lasts, the more chemical changes occur in the body, especially in the neuronal responses of the spinal cord, such that pain becomes harder to control. So do not wait until a person is screaming before administering pain medication; the objective is to eliminate all breakthrough pain. {See next chapter→Pain III.}

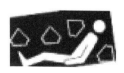

PAIN III

It may be difficult to convince the Departing to accept frequent doses of painkillers, especially opiates that are constipating, mind-fogging and sometimes nauseating. It used to be difficult to convince nurses and doctors to administer sufficient pain relief, since they had been trained to discourage addiction. It's now sometimes more difficult to convince patients, although the chance of addiction is statistically rare, and irrelevant during the Last Weeks or Days.

Eventually, there must be pain relief, and you must rely on laxatives and anti-emetics to manage the common side-effects. All painkillers have side-effects; opiates can cause frightening episodes of hallucination, →jerking, or slowed breathing.

These side-effects must be balanced against calibrations of pain, which are sometimes made using the McGill Pain Questionnaire, www.chcr.brown.edu/pcod/MCGILLPAINQUEST.PDF, but this requires the patient to be cogent. It is therefore inapt for people whose responsiveness has been compromised by stroke, paralysis, aphasia, opiates, or by pain itself. A better scale uses the contour of the lips (are they upturned, flat, twisted, or severely downturned?) and the openness of the →eyes (are they bright and open, somewhat narrowed, squinting under a furrowed brow, half-closed, or weeping, or tightly shut?) Here are some iconic shapes for the mouth/lips and what they may indicate with regard to degrees and dynamics of pain:

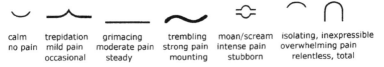

calm	trepidation	grimacing	trembling	moan/scream	isolating, inexpressible
no pain	mild pain	moderate pain	strong pain	intense pain	overwhelming pain
	occasional	steady	mounting	stubborn	relentless, total

Those who have bone pain, neuropathy, or other difficult-to-manage pain, may have a tiny pump inserted under the skin, with a →catheter going to the intrathecal space around the spinal cord. The pump automatically delivers a set amount of painkiller to the dorsal horn of the spine, so as to limit the number of pain messages sent to the brain and stimulate the release of natural opiates. Most pumps have an external switch by which to adjust the amount of painkiller.

It is a myth that the body becomes accustomed to opiates. If ever-higher dosages are needed, the pain itself is mounting, which is regularly the case, for example, with cancers that have metastasized to the bone.

No one wants to need to know any of this.

PAPERWORK

Skip this chapter, why don't you? I'd like to skip this chapter.
Here you are at the bedside during the Last Months or Weeks
or Days, or with family during the Days After, and all you want
to do is to be of help, or →grieve, and all you get is paperwork:

Last Months
Preparing or revising Advance →Directives, →wills, trusts.
Saving receipts for tax purposes, helping balance checkbooks.
Filling out intake forms for each new doctor, new hospital
Writing appeals to HMOs upon refusal of coverage.
Sending letters of inquiry to clinics, specialists.
Filling in patient histories on applications for drug trials.

Last Weeks/Days
Signing rental forms for medical equipment {→Doodads}.
Completing home health aide service forms.
Filling out →hospice assignment forms and contracts.

Days After
Filling out burial society or →funeral forms.
Composing →obituary notices for newspapers, newsletters.
Changing trusteeship in (or beneficiaries for) bank accounts.
Applying for life insurance or death benefits.

There is no avoiding this. Those at the bedside of the departing
poor may have fewer papers to deal with; they will never have
none. Even when departure itself is felt by all to be a relief,
there is little relief from repetitious paperwork. No one seems
to want to accept someone else's form with exactly the same
information. Every office wants its own form filled out
thoroughly. Widow/ers may even need to file two federal tax
forms and two state tax forms, the first as a couple filing jointly
for that part of the year during which moneys were coming to
both spouses, the second as an individual.

Paperwork should never devolve upon one person unless that
person has the time, inclination, and temperament--a rare
combination of patience, perseverance, delight in detail, and
good humor. If you hate paperwork, shout for →help. People
who hate paperwork do it poorly, and mistakes return to haunt
you. Paperwork is the most insistent of ghosts.

You might think that in this computerized, digitized world there
would be much less paperwork or forms to fill out online, where
mistakes are more easily remedied. Think again. Neither the
legal world nor the financial world nor the medical world trusts
the digital world, or "the cloud," when it comes to death and
dying. So paperwork still means *paper*work.

PARKING

Green Lot: Park as far as you can from the entrance to the hospital, hospice, or nursing home. If there are stairs, prefer them to elevators. This is all the exercise you are going to get while at the bedside, except for some pacing in corridors.

No joke. Legs can swell, arthritis flare up when you sit too long. If you just flew in and are rushing to the bedside {→Overnight Bags}, put some of that rush into jogging from far across the parking lot. Take the stairs down from the top of a parking structure, and back up again at the end of the day.

The fear is that you won't be there when the Departing needs you, or at the moment of departure {→ETD; Last Breaths}. But if your mind is cloudy and you are in some physical discomfort, you're not so much *present* as accountably there.

Those abed are not accountants of bodies. Your absence for twenty minutes to stretch your legs (and this means actively, athletically stretching) will not count against you. Back at the bedside, revived, you will be *present*.

Blue Lot: Whether you are walking or driving in a clinic lot or hospital parking structure, WATCH OUT: anxious, stressed people who have had little →sleep drive erratically or slowly and forget to use their turn signals. Twenty per cent of all driving accidents happen in parking lots. If drivers are rushing themselves or others to →Emergency, they are worse threats.

Red Lot: In our car culture, parking is also a euphemism for making out. Along with exercise, it's important to address another question of physicality at the bedside: holding hands. No, not holding hands with the Departing, but with your husband or →wife or fiancé(e) or lover. It may seem inappropriate, even a serious impropriety, in a hospital or hospice or household bedroom, to display any physical tenderness except toward the Departing: who's the focal point here, anyway? Don't you know that at a deathbed you're not supposed to be distracted by the romance in your own life when there is such sober asexual work at hand? {→Sex}

Yeah, making out at the bedside is a bit much, but holding hands is fine. The bedside demands more than spectatorship; invested as you are in being present, you cannot divest yourself of your own embodiment, your own needs for affection. A kiss, even a smooch, is not out of the question. For the Departing, seeing life go on is neither a tease nor a reprimand nor a flaunting of vitality. It's an assurance that when you are with them, you are who you always were. A friend, a parent, a lover.

PHARMACY & PHARMAKON {also→Medicines}

Pharmakon, in the Greek, refers both to a gift and a poison. So the history of medicine and of apothecaries teeters between cure and collapse. Our most powerful drugs can be the most deadly; an effective dose for one person can be fatal to another.

Be on guard, therefore, against mistakes in ordering, labeling, or addressing prescription drugs. And do consult with the pharmacist about drugs that work at cross-purposes with each other, or which may compound a problematic reaction.

As "controlled substances," opiates require special paperwork from doctors; such forms usually need to be hand-delivered to a pharmacy rather than faxed or called in. If the critically ill and Departing are not signed up with a →hospice that manages opiates internally, changes in controlled substance prescriptions can lead to puzzling delays as well as to denials or extra costs.

Health insurance companies and HMOs have formularies: lists of drugs that are covered at different tiers of co-payment. Some drugs may be available only by special request from your physician to a review board, or by personal appeal.

You can appeal denials. In cases where acute issues merit immediate action, an appeals process may take less than a week. Letters of denial usually tell you where and how to address an appeal. In a letter of appeal, include the following:
1. A concise description of the patient's current medical status;
2. The symptoms or pressing condition of urgent concern;
3. Your physician's argument as to why this drug/procedure is likely to be more effective (or produce less devastating side-effects) than others;
4. Citations from medical research (most easily accessible at www.ncbi.nlm.nih.gov/pubmed), demonstrating that the drug/procedure in question has been shown to be more effective than others typically prescribed;
5. A summary of all treatments already tried with no success;
6. A conclusion repeating your points: all other possibilities have been tried and found wanting; medical literature confirms that the drug/procedure at issue can help where all others have failed; suffering will be reduced and lifespan likely extended, if the drug/procedure works as it has in similar cases;
7. Appended: copies of letters in support of your appeal, signed by physicians. Send the letter by express mail, with tracking number and required signature.

Those who can afford to pay for expensive drugs/procedures on their own will not have to go through much of this.

PHYSICIANS AND SURGEONS

When Long Days become →Last Months, physicians will put in place the drugs and devices necessary for comfort, Except for broken limbs or food poisoning, no lab tests, x-rays, or scans will be scheduled. Aside from determining who will sign the death certificate, you may have little further to do with doctors.

The absence of physicians during the Last Days is striking--as though, no longer able to demonstrate their therapeutic mastery, physicians have left the building. And it is true: general practitioners and surgeons may see death all the time, but they do not see it as one of their prouder moments, while oncology nurses and pain specialists can take pride in their skill at easing a person toward departure. Understandably, many physicians recede from the bedside during the Last Days.

Historians have tried to pinpoint the times and places where the medical profession achieved such cultural ascendancy that death became unnatural--an event to be deplored as a failure of neurophysiological knowledge, pharmaceutical potency, and technological expertise. Death became unnatural in the late 1800s in Western Europe and the United States with the refinement of anaesthetics and aseptic procedures, the advent of bacteriology, and campaigns for vaccination. Held at bay in ways that made its clutch on the living seem negotiable, death (except war death) was increasingly "unexpected." The earlier the death, the more unnatural it was, since ostensibly more preventable through better medicine, nutrition, and programs for infant care and public health.

Some people do rise from their deathbeds, against all odds, only to die four or five months later: they still had work to do, →anniversaries to reach. A remarkable few beat the odds entirely and rise from their deathbeds to live for years in good health. Physicians will look up from their laptops, surprised--surprised, though not necessarily pleased. After all, they are the premier oddsmakers, and it is their odds-making that makes a "miraculous" recovery appear miraculous.

Historical epidemiology reveals that neither medical nor surgical advances put humanity on its course toward longer life. It was better sanitation and a still-inexplicable cycling down of epidemic diseases. Although individuals may owe their longer lives to a new drug or procedure, as an aggregate we live longer for other, more non-specific, reasons. During the Last Days we die, or live on to other Last Days, for reasons that have little to do with physicians and surgeons. They may still be on-call, but their calling lies elsewhere.

PLAIN PINE BOXES

Coffinmakers of Ghana delight in crafting wooden airplanes and limousines for the Departed, who in their lives never flew, never went first class. There is no rule that a coffin be somber or soundproof.

The wishes of the Departed are rarely as solid and sober as those of the owners of funeral parlors and managers of burial grounds, for whom good taste and grand ceremony are quite profitable. The Departing are always more interested in the liveliness of a memorial service than in the tonnage of a monument, and have more to say about the songs to be sung at a wake than the style of inscription on a stone.

Under the pressures of →grief and guilt, of wanting to do right by the Departed in the haste of the Days After, one is ever in jeopardy of doing violence to the tenor of the departure or the wishes of the Departing. The burial may be for the Departed and for the Health Department, but the memorial service, procession, stone, and inscription are for those who will be around to read, to speak, to weep, to walk the sharp-mown aisles of a cemetery.

A recent movement among observant Jews has reasserted the rabbinic dictum that it suffices for all to be buried in plain pine boxes. Everywhere now, catering to most religious traditions, you can find cooperative burial societies that establish base rates well under a thousand dollars for a simple coffin and burial, or a green burial (with a biodegradable casket, shroud, or blanket), or cremation and urn, or the scattering of ashes at sea. One can also have ashes sealed in a mortuary crypt or buried in a family plot. (Warning: If just one family member is present at the graveside during the burial of ashes, this may qualify as a graveside service and a cemetery can charge you hundreds of dollars more.)

Is it perverse to suggest to the Departing that friends and family may take joy in the departure, if it be a release from pain and terrible confusion? Is it wrong to suggest that people may be enheartened by a departure in which a death is subsumed by the recounting of the lovingkindness of a life? No.

Coffins, caskets, and their optional features need not be encumbrances upon death. Plain pine boxes are hardly a disgrace, nor are ceremonies without rich trappings. It is not the body that must live on.

POLITICS AND STRANGE BEDSIDES

Just a century ago, few arrived at adulthood without having lost a brother or sister. Infant mortality was high: two in every ten infants died before their first birthday. Childhood mortality was almost as high, due to infectious diseases in crowded cities, against which there were as yet no antibiotics and no effective codes against shoddily-built tenements and sewage lines. Early deaths resulted as well from severe nutritional deficits, against which there were as yet neither isolated vitamins nor effective ordinances against adulterated milk. Life expectancy was compromised in the long run by lung disorders, for which there were as yet the weakest of pollution laws against smoke (let alone against smoking), while some physicians insisted that the carbon and sulfur of industrial smoke invigorated the lungs.

And given that maternal mortality at childbirth was also high, by the time that a person born in 1900 reached the age of 30, s/he would likely have been to a funeral for a mother or father as well as a brother or sister.

This is not counting war or murder.

Infant mortality in the United States remains inexcusably high-- higher than in thirty-five other countries. Maternal mortality is higher than in twenty-seven other countries. In murders per capita, the U.S. ranks twenty-fourth among sixty-two countries. Nonetheless, overall average life expectancy at birth is 78, much higher than in 1900, though lower than in Japan, Italy, Israel, Australia, Macau, and thirty other nations.

What's the point of this exercise in numbers? First, that politics and economics, the making of law and making of profits, have a considerable, measurable role to play in the production of Long Days. Second, that we are nowhere near as familiar with bedsides as were our great-grandparents and grandparents. Reading their diaries and letters, you would find that our ancestors were not stoics about death or brusque with the dying. However, they lived in communities more accustomed to death watches and preparations for death.

Politics and economics have much to do with how young they die, good food and clean air with how long and how well they live. In the run-up to the Last Days, you may vow to devote yourself to a cause that will reduce the mortality from cancer, heart disease, diabetes, or fight against automatic weapons, industrial toxins, irresponsible financiers. During the Last Days, however, the bedside is not really yours: it is the common ground between you and the Departing. Strangers come later.

POWER OF ATTORNEY

Power of Attorney, as distinct from a Durable Power of Attorney for Health Care, refers to a formal, usually notarized document that gives another person or persons the legal (proxy) authority to manage one's assets, including all bank accounts, stocks, pension income, and real estate holdings. Power of Attorney can be assigned to a spouse, an adult child, a relative, a friend, a family lawyer; ordinarily an alternate is named as well. The person(s) designated as having Power of Attorney may or may not also have Durable Power of Attorney for Health Care.

Those who have set up trusts will already have Power of Attorney documents in their trust packet. Copies should be kept at home in a fireproof safe or vault, in each set of emergency papers, and (where available) in a safe deposit box.

Someone exercising Power of Attorney is supposed to pay all bills and to allocate remaining resources on behalf of a person who cannot manage his own financial affairs due to injury, illness, or mental deterioration. If and when a person recovers, all rights to manage her affairs return to her, and she can at any time cancel or change the assignment of Power of Attorney.

Power of Attorney financial issues often cross paths with the issues of Durable Power of Attorney for Health Care. If a person seeks out an experimental treatment {→Risk} that is not covered by insurance, then a calculation of costs and benefits will be vital to both the financial and health care proxies. So too for deciding upon a homecare agency. If hired →caregivers appear to be exploiting those in their care and receiving expensive gifts from them, both sets of proxies may have to intervene. So it is best if the person(s) acting with Power of Attorney and Durable Power of Attorney for Health Care are on good terms with each other.

Power of Attorney ends with death. This is important. At death, the directives of a →will take precedence, even with regard to the paying of bills. An estate worth over a certain trigger limit (different in each state) must go through probate unless a prior Trust has been established. Once triggered, and regardless of the existence of a will, a state Probate Court determines the sequence through which an estate's wealth will be distributed: to estate administrators, funeral expenses, and creditors first, before heirs. The probate process can be lengthy and tedious.

Heads up: I suspect that every line on this page could be challenged in court, where large figures are at stake. My summary here has no legal standing.

PRE-EXISTING CONDITIONS

Bugaboo of many who have sought and bought health insurance, the pre-existing conditions clause for (private-pay) major medical coverage will be eliminated with the full implementation of the Affordable Health Care Act as signed into law by President Obama on March 23, 2010, and upheld by the Supreme Court on June 28, 2012.

But the Act does not entirely eliminate pre-existing conditions clauses. All those on Medicare who, *after* the expiration of their Initial Enrollment Period at age 65, seek to add supplemental (Medigap) insurance can be subject to the rigors of medical underwriting--determination of insurability--when subsequently seeking Medigap coverage.

Restated: Anyone who initially signed up for Medicare Part A (hospital, nursing) and Part B (visits to doctors, medical equipment) **only** and who desires to add Medigap insurance more than six months later may be susceptible to underwriting. Even upon issuing an acceptance, insurers may insert a pre-existing conditions clause that exempts them from reimbursing any expenses incurred (e.g.) during the first 3 months of coverage that hearken back to conditions treated in the last 3 months before coverage began.

Exception: if a person enrolls in a Medicare Advantage Plan during the Initial Enrollment Period and then switches to a Medigap plan during the annual Open Enrollment Period (~October 15-~December 7), no underwriting determinations are required and no pre-existing conditions clause can be inserted.

There are numerous other exceptions and provisos: see www.medicare.gov/Pubs/pdf/11219.pdf.

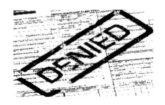

PRE-EXISTING CONDITIONS, continued

Of course, we all have pre-existing conditions. A building inspector for a program of grants to low-income homeowners once assured me that "incipient decay" was a valid reason for applying for funds for house improvements. Across the heavens as on Earth, what is not subject to incipient decay? Over billions of years, the very stars will blink out. Our bodies are far more finite. If for all practical purposes it's not true that we begin dying the moment we're born, it is true that apoptosis, cell death, is inherent to our living, and few of us escape the more visible, external signs of decay as we age.

So the seriously ill, with the collusion of those at the bedside, may scrutinize their lives with an eye to hidden processes and autobiographical, familial, or genetic origins of disease and frailty. Those bedridden as the result of serious→accident may still try to puzzle out why things keep happening to them.

And so we say that "her smoking finally caught up with him," or "he had it coming, he was always a reckless driver," or "didn't we tell her that she'd end up a basket case if she didn't get out more, eat better, take vitamins." As if an illness or Departure were time's inevitable revenge, the mean momentum of incipient decay.

Yet here we sit, at the bedside, caught up in the same mean momentum, getting dehydrated. Are we in denial? Isn't something bound to happen to us? Something working its way through our systems, unseen, unheralded?

Whoa. Get off your duff, go for a walk, get a drink of water, write a real letter. For some billions of years, the world will go on with or without you. Right now, which is it to be?

PREPARING THE BODY

For each one who departs by land, three or four depart by sea.

This is a metaphor of the texture, smell, and sound of dying.

Less often than any would wish, departures are clean. The Departing looks wan but presentable, speaks softly but intelligibly. The skin has been washed, hair brushed, earwax removed, →teeth flossed, →nails clipped, →hands and feet smoothed with lotion. Call this a departure by land: dry, stable, approachable.

More often than any would wish, departures are a mess. The Departing looks absent or wild-eyed, →speaks in bubbles or punctuates the awful effort of breathing with words half-vowel, half-spit. There is →pain in lying still, and the skin is afire. A bedbath is out of the question. The mouth is rank with the smell of drugs or the dry blood of a bitten →tongue. Abdomen and ankles are swollen. Call this a departure by sea: wet, stormy, off-putting.

Most Last Days are amphibian, neither so staunch as by land nor so nauseous as by sea. One must be prepared for both.

This is not a page about how to prepare a body for burial but about preparing yourself for the physical changes in a person who is dying. In some traditions, laypeople lay out the body; regardless of tradition or training, all of us are laypeople when it comes to facing up to the body of the →Last Days.

The more dramatic the physical changes, the more you try to convince yourself that whatever is not body remains intact {→Accidentals}. However, there may be incoherencies of word and mind, outbursts of anger or profanity so uncharacteristic that you keep having to shake off the idea that the person you knew is no longer around but has departed ahead of the body, which, left to itself, is making a clumsy, graceless exit.

To be blunt: preparing yourself for a body in such flux is no harder than managing the body of an infant or small child all of whose orifices must be cared for almost hourly, and whose inevitable fevers, ear infections, and teething are more painful than you can remember. (Is this why we forget our earliest years?) The difference, and difficulty, with the Departing is that the preparations seem so unrewarding or unnecessary. It is after all only a body {→Identity}. But when does one ever say such a thing to oneself or to another, except under torture or in the Last Days? Until the end we all need lanterns, though we find few wise men, more wise women.

p.r.n.

Pro re nata: as circumstances arise, taken by pharmacists, nurses, and doctors to mean "use as needed."

It may be on the labels of rescue inhalers for asthmatics and bottles of morphine drops for those in the Last Months. Often, *p.r.n.* has limits, as with the number of times a day that one should use a rescue inhaler, or as with acetaminophen (not more than 3000-4000 mg in a 24-hour period, and lower if simultaneously taking Percocet or Roxilox, because these are compounds of oxycodone and acetaminophen; or when also taking Norco, Vicodin, Anexsia, Liquicet, Lorcet, Lortab, Maxidone, Polygesic, Xodol, Zamicet, Zolvit, Zydone, because these are compounds of hydrocodone and acetaminophen.)

Simple enough: *p.r.n.* puts the timing and frequency of the use of →medications squarely in the hands of patients. What freedom! What a sense of security! He can use this whenever he wants, I can get it for her whenever she asks. No hand-wringing, no trying to reach a doctor after hours. It's *p.r.n.*

In practice, however, *p.r.n.* often means, "We can't predict everything, so it's up to you," and "Don't blame us if things go haywire."

Exactly what circumstances could arise, do arise? You must ask that question and get answers that make sense. Will there be occasions when the patient will not know to ask, or be too weak or weak-voiced to ask, or too confused, agitated, nauseous? Will there be times when it should not be given even when directly asked for? Who decides, and how?

"As needed," then, is not synonymous with "as circumstances arise." In daily life, unique circumstances always arise, yet we are slow to adjust our needs. Needs are more conservative than circumstances. Are you--you at the bedside--now the arbiter between needs and circumstances?

Consider →pain. Those in pain should call the shots, but even in hospice many hesitate to call for painkillers when they first feel pain. They have their reasons: they don't want to become "addicted"; they fear that overuse of painkillers will reduce their effectiveness in future, even more painful episodes;. But once a person is in pain, the body is in stress, and so are the bodies and minds of those at the bedside. Avoiding or delaying painkillers weakens all systems, including the system of care. What does *p.r.n.* mean now? "Use when not needed"?

QUALITY OF LIFE

Quality of life issues are, well, qualitative. Some dubiously quantitative scales have been proposed, but they are, well, dubious. Trained rather as scientists than ethicists, physicians tend to be uneasy when it comes to calculations of desire, discomfort, and despondency. So when medicine begins to appear, to its own practitioners, intrusive or daredevil, "quality of life" comes to the fore, and physicians disengage themselves from the foggiest or most conflicted aspects of a situation.

To be fair, when quality of life issues arise during the Long Days with regard to neurosurgeries, amputations, stem cell transplants, and kidney dialysis, teams of physicians, nurses, and →social workers do forthrightly discuss with patients the short- and long-term →risks and consequences of embracing, deferring, or refraining from a grave procedure or (lifelong) treatment.

In many other circumstances, quality of life issues are not broached until there remains just one issue, quality of death, in which case "quality of life" is rather a medical euphemism that allows for the finessing of responsibility.

Why the uneasiness? The shedding of responsibility? Don't physicians make life-or-death decisions every day in emergency rooms, operating rooms? Or are decisions about quality of life as much on behalf of the caregivers as of the Departing? Isn't it pleasanter for those at the bedside to bear witness to a relatively painless, quiet, unchallenging departure?

Where quality of life comes to the fore as neither the gambit of physicians nor the cloaked wishes of those at the bedside, then perhaps it should be understood as an expression of things that we do not ever want to give up on. The serious ill and the Departing, don't they have rights to liberty, equity, respect? If we become cynical, won't that undermine our own notions about how life should be lived at all times, balancing work, play, self, and family, personal success and collective altruism, →urgency and history? What if the variables we have used for decades to assess our own quality of life are now irrelevant?

When oncologists, surgeons, internists, or hospice staff say that the time has come to consider quality of life, make no mistake: they are not giving you guidance, nor are they posing a chess problem in end-games. They are asking you to rethink the criteria by which, in earlier years, life meant something more than smoothly working bodily functions. . . or to reconceive life as little more than bodily and mental functions that unravel as smoothly and painlessly as possible. How much more, exactly?

QUESTIONING

<u>On Questioning Physicians</u>
Priding themselves on being in the know, physicians (above all, specialists) dislike being presented with print-outs from recent research of which they are unaware. Unless part of a research unit, they respond blandly to published reports of positive results from recent trials. Although prognoses of a year or less{→ETD} would seem to be a cue to seek out experimental therapies, physicians often want to wait for more evidence, more scientific confirmation. Options you suggest after much research they may therefore dismiss as grasping at straws. You mean to be acting staunchly; they make you feel like an impetuous fool, willing to drag the Departing through hell and high water to prove your everlasting love or a new medical theory. You must in turn be resolute in questioning them.

Ask about:
Operating assumptions:
---What's your best guess as to what's going on?
---What don't you know? What else could be going on?
---Is this one disease or could it be several running in tandem?
Implications of various treatments or approaches:
---What may be the cognitive and emotional side-affects?
---Which are synergistic (more effective in combination)?
---Which are home-based, which require treatment centers?
Familial consequences:
---Does this have a genetic component or cause sterility?
---What is the bearing on the lives of children or siblings?

<u>On Questioning Bureaucrats</u> (Insurance, Hospital, SNF)
Everybody at a desk wants to believe they're doing the best they can to help you, or that rules from above prevent that. They'll apologize for delays but not for mistakes made at other levels, so you must be prepared to repeat your story to echelon after echelon before your questions are fully answered, your logic taken seriously. Treat each person with respect, but keep records of all conversations, with names and dates, and never change your story. Where you are challenging a decision or seeking a policy exception, be sure to write down your story, questions, and issues beforehand. It's sometimes best to begin each conversation with a confession of confusion; this allows the people across a desk from you, or on the phone, to feel competent, because there are things they can tell you that you're unlikely to know. Sometimes this itself leads to a satisfactory resolution. If not, stay the course without threatening anyone, all the while repeating your story and keeping records that can support legal action {→lawyers}.

QUID PRO QUO

Whoever raised you--parents, grandparents, aunts, uncles--don't you owe them the years of care that they took in seeing you safely from infancy to maturity? Isn't there a *quid pro quo* that draws you to the bedside for as long as you are wanted?

You squirm. After all, you didn't *ask* to be born, didn't *ask* to be fed and housed for however many years. Isn't it a kind of →blackmail when someone who voluntarily raised you demands your presence at the bedside for weeks at a time?

But they didn't *ask* to be ill, or bedridden or palsied. . . . You might think (and say?) that their salty fatty diet, their lack of exercise, their smoking has finally done them in and you've been warning them for years, right? about diabetes, heart attacks, emphysema, lung disease, strokes, colon cancer--and guess what's happened, guess what?, so why should you come running to their bedside now?

Look who's talking! Remember how stubborn you were as a kid, getting into all kinds of scrapes and falling sick with the mumps fourteen times, and it certainly isn't their fault that they got this sclerosis or rare blood disease, and maybe you have it in your genes too. Who's going to take care of you when, as they say, the gene "expresses" itself?

You've taken care of yourself, in all ways, since you were a teen, and if they'd only gone to see the specialist when you asked them to, they wouldn't need you or anyone else to suffer with them through this newest crisis, you have a family too, sons and daughters you love, but that's neither here nor there since you physically can't be both here and there.

What do you know about love? They gave up their careers to raise you, worked three jobs, had golden opportunities, once-in-a-lifetime chances, but you were always more important, your health, your schooling, your happiness, and now that they're sick you begrudge them a couple of months? When they're gone, you know, they've set aside something for the grandkids, there'll be →money for them to become bigshots.

Then use the money now to hire →caregivers, you'll help *them*.

What, and invite strangers into the house? The house you grew up in? Shame on you. Better they should kick the bucket tomorrow. No, this afternoon. They'll make an appointment this afternoon . . . and this one they'll keep.

Quid pro quo.

QUID PRO QUO, IN REVERSE

We can take care of ourselves. We raised you and your
→brothers and sisters and when you had all made lives for
yourselves, we made another life for ourselves, a decent life,
moving out of the old house into a smaller place, managing our
finances so none of you ever had to support us. That was our
goal, no one should ever have the burden of supporting two
→generations, the past and the future. So you get on with
your lives and we'll get on with ours. Why are you here at our
bedsides when you should be with your wife, husband, kids,
job? The old make way for the young, that's how it is. We
have Medicare, we even have Medigap; when it's necessary
we'll go into assisted living, into a nursing home, into one of
those "memory units," wherever, (→SNF},don't worry about us.

But I want to be here. I owe it to you. You've done so much
for me, gone out of your way, and I *liked* the old house, all you
needed was a cleaning service and a gardener, I could easily
have arranged for that, and maid service now, or a handyman
to install some safety bars in the bathroom. I'll pay for it all,
it's not a problem, and look, I bought some smoke alarms to
put up in the kitchen and bedroom, and I put new batteries in
your remotes and your flashlights. I just want you to be safe
and secure and happy and back to health and I'm here to help.
What do you need?

Really, we don't need anything. That →fall we took, everyone
slips now and then, maybe we'll get rid of the throw rugs from
around the place and we promise we'll use our →walkers more,
even from room to room, OK? You can go home now, you must
be tired from those hours in emergency, in the hospital, and
we're keeping you from your business, your books, your family.
You got us these bracelets with the beeper things so even if we
do fall, everyone this side of Antarctica will know about it and
firemen and ambulances will appear in a flash. So go. Go.

Are you sure? I could cook some meals to put in the freezer.
I've set up your meds for the week, but I could buy one of
those monster pill holders and fill it for the whole month. And
what about the visiting nurse? Who's taking you to your
doctor's appointment next Tuesday? Do you want me to see
about that dripping faucet in the bathtub?

What dripping faucet? You're hearing things. Listen, if we
need you we'll call you. You can't be spending so much time
with us, it's a blessing, but you don't owe us anything.

I owe you everything. Maybe I'll stay a few more days.

READINESS

Whose?

The synchronicities of the bedside are humanly imperfect. Sometimes the Departing is ready for the departure long before those at the bedside; sometimes, though they may not admit it, those at the bedside are ready for the departure long before the Departing. Sometimes one side of the family is ready, another side not. Or friends, and not the family.

This is no one's fault. Even →wives and husbands who have been together for fifty years may continue to move through life at different rhythms, and depart at distinct tempi.

The reasons that the Departing may hang back from death can be simple: someone still to arrive; a personal deadline or →anniversary. Or the Departing may be waiting for someone at the bedside to be reconciled to departure: a last kindness.

The reasons that the Departing may rush toward death can also be simple:→pain; great →fatigue; fear of losing whatever grasp on reality remains; fear of becoming a financial drain on the family as "a vegetable." Well, no, these are not so simple.

Some at the bedside may refuse to be reconciled to a departure if it is thought to be premature, unjust, or the result of medical malpractice {→Iatrogenesis}. If a departure comes on the heels of another equally grievous departure, it is hard not to feel at once shocked and furious, feelings that can lead to an unusual obstinacy ("I will not allow this to happen--again") or to an anger that is misdirected at the Departing ("How can you do this to me now? Why couldn't you have held on for another year and given me some time to heal from the first death?")

Those who have been reconciled to the departure for months may feel guilty that they've done their mourning prematurely. With their carefully-won equanimity, are they to blame for a departure that's come too soon for others, or for the Departing --as if they'd hurried Death? {→Holding On.}

The guilt, shock, anger, remorse must all be talked through in Days After. What can be expressed immediately is permission to depart. Family and friends who see the Departing struggling to stay on, despite pain and utter fatigue, can take up the hand of the Departing, or gently press a palm to the →breastbone, and tell him it's OK to go, tell her there's no need to linger.

READING

Enforced stillness in a comfortable bed with good light: on first thought that would seem conducive to reading. Every once in a while, don't you yourself consider locking the doors, shutting off the →cell phone, and declaring yourself "dead to the world" so as to get through all the books and papers stacking up?

Dying, it turns out, is not a good time for catching up on your reading. Nor is illness when painful, feverish, debilitating. But those at the bedside will need several sorts of books at hand: a book to read silently to oneself in quiet times; a book worthy of being read aloud; a book in reserve to read to young children.

Well-written books help us shape our thoughts by modeling syntax, rhythm, tone, meaning, and the give-and-take of good conversation. They are encouragements to mutual →reflection as well as to private meditation. They take time seriously even as they lift the reader out of one time into another.

I'm not talking about escapist fiction. Hospital janitors must toss a hundred potboilers into the compactor or furnace every night. It's misguided to choose a book that you can read mindlessly and leave off at any moment. You need a book that you enjoy reading slowly and whose passages you circle because you want to read them to others. The time you spend at the bedside is for savoring, whether in lively company during the Long Days or while the Departing→sleeps.

It's difficult to study at any bedside, even at home, but to enter into a fiction is entirely possible. Why? Perhaps it is because fictions have conclusions, final pages that are culminating pages even when they allow for diverse interpretations. Following a life closely to its end is not unlike following a novel to its ending. A story is incomplete without an end, and although a good story may end tragically, its end has been well-prepared, so that it is meaningful and fits within a logic that began building from the first page. One hopes that one's own departure will have a similar meaningfulness, however subject it may be to a host of interpretations. One wants to have done enough to allow for richness of interpretation, and one wants to die at the right point along the curve of the tale.

Of course, few have the control over their lives that a novelist has over her characters, over his confluences of event and person. But imagine finishing the last sentence of the last paragraph of a novel moments before the →Last Words....

RECYCLING

I volunteer at a Community Resource Center that has thrift stores and a food pantry. Every week we receive donations from families in which someone has died.

Health regulations dictate that we immediately discard the following: open cartons or bags of food and spices; long-expired cans and bottles of food; open tubes or jars of toiletries and cosmetics; open packages of foot plasters and bandages; used combs, brushes, and razors; cookbooks crusted with pie dough. If you bring these to us (really, dump these on us), we must toss them, and incur a hefty waste disposal fee each month. Offer such items to friends, neighbors, and relatives, or dump them in your own garbage.

That said, much else can and should be recycled through senior centers, non-profit groups, or local, national, or international charities. For example:

++First Aid
unopened packages of dressings, bandages, band-aids, gauze,
    plasters, moleskin, wipes, cotton swabs, washcloths
metal scissors and nail clippers, so long as not rusty;
over-the-counter (and unused) antibiotic ointments, lotions.

++Medical appliances: {→Doodads}
canes
commodes (unused)
emesis basins (unused)
grabbers
Hoyer lifts
pill boxes, pill cutters (gently used);
shower hand bars or rails, toilet bars or rails
sippy cups (unused)
walkers
wheelchair lifts or attachments for vans and cars
wheelchairs, standard or electric

++Beds, Bedding, Toiletries
adult diapers (packages unopened)
bed mirrors
bedsteads
feminine hygiene pags (packages unopened)
mattresses: alternating pressure vinyl mattresses are OK
    but health regulations preclude accepting standard or foam
    mattresses. They also preclude house slippers, false teeth.
pillows: only if unused
sheets, if unstained and washed thoroughly

RECYCLING, continued

++Prescription Medicines:

In the past it was illegal to recycle prescription drugs within the United States, but since 2003 Nebraska, Wisconsin, Colorado, Ohio, and Minnesota have created drug repository programs where individuals as well as health care facilities can donate unexpired, sealed medications for redistribution in-state to needy patients with cancer and serious chronic or terminal illnesses. Other states (Illinois, Missouri, Maryland, Georgia) are contemplating such programs. Meanwhile, it is legal for humanitarian agencies, such as Aid for AIDS or Child Family Health International, to send unexpired, unopened prescription medicines to countries whose citizens have little or no access to expensive drugs. Ask your community health clinic about options in your region. {→Medicine Cabinets, Medicines }

Medicines that cannot be donated should not be flushed down the toilet, lest the chemicals enter our waterways; they should be disposed of as household hazardous waste. Each locale has sites for hazardous waste disposal.

++Wigs, scarves, hats, and specialty bras:

Cancer patients often have a wardrobe of morale-boosting garments and accessories that will be accepted and thoroughly cleaned by hospice organizations and some commercial shops devoted to helping those undergoing chemotherapy and radiation.

++Electronics:

CD players
→Cell phones
walkie-talkies
reading lamps,
assistive devices for the hard-of-hearing and visually impaired.

Computers are not so easily recycled, especially monitors (which contain toxic mercury), but some service organizations recycle these without a fee. Do not dump old monitors or glitch-ridden, broken, or outmoded computers (including laptops, notebooks, tablets) on thrift stores; they will end up having to pay for disposal or recycling.

REFLECTION

Among the small, unanticipated changes during the Last Days: the disappearance of mirrors. Woman or man, the Departing has less and less interest in using a mirror.

Seeing the complexion go pale, the cheeks and eye sockets go hollow, the skin become taut but dry, you may also be reluctant to produce a pocket mirror for the application of make-up.

You may think to use a pocket mirror for another purpose: to assure yourself that a person is still breathing during scary periods of apnea or →aspiration.   In this case, what you are looking for is neither clarity nor perspective but fog. Fog as an index to life. . . .*There* is cause for reflection.

And consider also the mirror-like reflections off →windows at certain times of day. In these moments you see yourself and the Departing reflected together but askew or fragmented, oddly framed by ledges and the edges of shutters or blinds. Should we call these glimpses an omen?

Mirrors shimmer between the literal and the figurative, blatancy and reversal. In many cultures, the family at departure covers over the mirrors throughout the house, lest the soul of the Departing become transfixed in the glass. Whatever mirrors tell us about ourselves, whatever we behold in them, they also somehow threaten to withhold: glasses half empty and half full.

Vanity is not the issue here. The issue is the nature of communion at the bedside during the Last Days. Do you try to hold up a mirror to the Departing, let her see herself in your eyes as she needs now to see herself, let him make peace with the person he has become? Or do you reflect on the past, individually and jointly, in an effort to come to terms with a life almost spent? Do you serve as a handheld mirror or as a full-length portable mirror on wheels or rollers, the kind of mirror once known technically as a *psyche*.

Technical caution: standard mirrors reverse from side to side, not top to bottom. The physics of this is no less complicated than the psychology.

All of us, by the by, are asymmetrical, in body as in life.

RESPITE

Respite these days has become something of a technical term, referring to relief for caregivers.

→Hospices, presuming that someone will be attending upon the Departing 24 hours a day, provide respite volunteers for 9-12 hours a week. These volunteers have been trained to sit at the bedside and chat with the Departing, read to them, do cooking or light housecleaning while the Departing is asleep, but they cannot administer medicines or change dressings. Should a medical problem arise while you are away or getting some well-earned sleep, they will immediately call a hospice nurse.

Cancer, multiple sclerosis, Parkinson's, and AIDS networks in your area may provide supplementary respite. The ARCH National Respite Coalition's website, www.respitelocator.org, lists state respite coalitions, some of whom provide respite through unpaid volunteers, some through contracts with for-profit home health aide/caregiver →agencies.

For those during the Long Days who are frail of mind and body but otherwise in stable health, many day centers are opening up. Some can be located through the National Group Respite Program at www.brookdalefoundation.org/respiteprogram.htm and others through state or county departments of ageing. "Eldercare" is a new keyword through which you may find local not-for-profit and for-profit respite assistance.

Of course, you can also ask →friends or other family members to sit in for you, with instructions to call the doctor's office or hospice if anything arises to which they feel inadequate. This is not workable in the long run because weekly schedules are complicated, health problems among friends and neighbors get in the way, and some family members are squeamish about being at the bedside as the responsible person.

The point is that caregivers at home need →help, and part of that help must come in the form of respite. An exhausted, blurry-eyed, dehydrated caregiver can jeopardize pain control, wound care, and general equilibrium. Even if the bedside is in a →SNF or hospital, you may need respite--time to sleep, shower, answer messages, keep family and friends informed, pay your bills, water the plants.

No one will begrudge you these intervals for recuperation. The ill and Departing will not blame you if they wake to someone else at the bedside. They do not keep count of the number of hours you have been absent from the bedside. And let's be honest, they may need some respite from you.

A blank page. Not absolutely blank, and neither transparent nor weightless.

This is respite. You may do what you want with the blankness, but you do not vanish. You are away from the bedside, but you are not absent from all that is substantial. Blankness, like this page, is an opening. It is not emptiness.

RICTUS

Pick-up by a mortuary or cremation society is not immediate. Once notified, it will be an hour or more before their van arrives.

(If the departure takes place in a →skilled nursing facility, a board-and-care, or a retirement home, the staff will make the call, as predesignated, and the mortuary or cremation society will in turn notify the coroner; if the departure takes place at home under →hospice care, you will notify hospice, who will in turn make all the arrangements. In either case, the coroner is not going to come.)

Sometimes the Departing close their →eyes before they die; sometimes they do not. Ordinarily, they do not tell you that they are about to go, nor do they press your hand or blink one last time, or turn away {→Last Breaths}.

Often, however, in the hour(s) during which you may still be in the room awaiting the van, their faces relax into a small smile. They do not become instantly cold, so for a while the smile remains warm.

That lingering smile is the result of rictus, the settling of muscles in the face. If the skin is tight, the smile may become a grin, and if the lips are slightly parted, as sometimes they are, then the grin may look menacing or antic.

Morticians have methods for smoothing out the features into a generic calm, mouth closed. But you will be in the presence of a face that is apparently more active, more meaningful. You may be dressing the body in the clothes requested, or →sitting quietly, or calling family and friends, or cleaning up around the room. Whatever you are doing, the smile of the Departed may come to feel particularly disconcerting, even eerie.

One would be surprised by the number of cases in which Departed women appear to be smiling like the Mona Lisa, enigmatic yet engaging. What are they thinking?

Neurological and neuromuscular disorders may make the rictus of a smile impossible, as may death while in extreme pain. Death does not demand or solicit a smile after the Last Days. But when it does happen, it can be reassuring. It is almost impossible not to look for meaning in that smile, and find it.

RISK

Sigrid Fry-Revere, in an opinion piece for the *Los Angeles Times* (16 August 2007), criticized the Court of Appeals for the District of Columbia for ruling that "terminally ill patients do not have a constitutional right to use experimental treatments without being enrolled in a clinical trial . . . even if their doctors believe that such treatment is their best chance for survival." She argued that this "safety first" principle is neither kind nor helpful. When given a prognosis {→ETD} and apprised of the limited chance that something new may help, the terminally ill can make rational choices. They should not be blocked from receiving treatment because all the data are not in, or because an "unacceptable" percentage of test patients die.

During the →Last Months and weeks, the ill and the Departing may have applications outstanding for experimental drug trials or new protocols. They may be vocal about trying unorthodox treatments, flying to a clinic in Mexico or Myanmar, importing non-traditional healers, or drinking herbal extracts labeled in unfamiliar characters. They may decide to fast. They may make detailed plans for an exotic go-for-broke vacation.

Should you aid in these efforts because they are welcome evidence of a never-say-die activism? Or must you be the voice of reason, which can sound like the voice of doom?

Let's figure this out.

At the bedside a person is obliged to five things:
   1. attentiveness;
   2. an affectionate steadiness;
   3. immediate practical help;
   4. knowledge of the current diet, regime of medications, and schedule of treatments;
   5. astute anticipation of needs.

You may also want to be sensitive to moods and to side-effects of drugs that alter mood, but you are not obliged to share ambitions, schemes, or dreams, nor are you obliged to agree at all times with the Departing.

For any given scheme or dream, you should listen well, offer up pros and cons, suggest avenues of recourse--in other words, participate in a conversation. Afterwards, if you judge a scheme to be ill-advised, say so, plainly but without the use of demeaning or defeatist language {→Frankness}.

RISK, continued

Here are some questions that can be kind and helpful in making decisions about taking treatment →risks at turning points on the path toward (or maybe away from) departure:

---What do you need to do that cannot be accomplished in the time supposed to remain? Can I help you finish up, or must you do it on your own?

---Will a longer life mean a more painful or narcotized life than is already the case?

---What are you willing to give up in order to live on? What not?

Then there are questions less kind, and far more awkward to pose:

---If the cost of experimental medicines or procedures is likely to be such as nearly to bankrupt the family {→Money}, is the promise of a somewhat longer life worth risking the financial well-being of those who will live on afterward?

---If the cost of the medicines or procedures will be borne by the government, but at such expense that other services provided by the State must be reduced, at what time in the consideration of personal risk and benefit must one take into ethical account the health of the commonweal?

Questions of risk inevitably abut issues of selfishness and →quality of life. When you gamble on life and death, who else is in the game? What *is* the game?

ROOMMATES

Hospice facilities ordinarily have single rooms, but in hospitals and nursing homes most of the Departing share a semi-private room with a roommate who is not about to die. The roommate may be coughing continually, moaning, snoring, or breathing with such difficulty that s/he seems to be on the verge of collapse, but that sense of a mutual departure is due to the pathos of the situation, in which you are at the bedside of someone approaching death only to be disturbed by a person in the same room struggling mightily to live.

And there are strange people coming and going at the bedside of the roommate, trying hard to be respectful of the thin curtain separating the two patients, yet audible, felt presences. And they are not talking about death but about work, business, family, the damnable food, days before discharge.

Meanwhile you and the Departing are working on resolution, maybe even an →obituary. It's tempting to begin thinking like the visitors on the other side, who discuss second chances and returns to normality. Or, vice versa, to be thankful that the Departing is not in such pain, yet wondering whether the acute pain audible from the other side would be worth it if there were a chance of another two or three months {→Quality of Life}.

Sometimes the roommate and the Departing become friends, and the curtain opens. Sometimes the roommates are too transient, upset, alienated, →grumpy or confused to become friends. On a few occasions, the visitors and those at the bedside of the Departing also become friendly.

What do you say to →friends and visitors who know that one bed is a last resting place, the other not?

What do all of you make of the discomfiting circumstance of sharing a room day after day with a stranger or a rotating set of strangers at a time like this, when having a roommate likely hearkens back to experiences almost forgotten and decades ago as a child at overnight camp, or a college student in a dormitory, or a soldier in military quarters? How does this haphazard, enforced sharing of close quarters affect the very nature of our modern notions of illness and dying? A good topic for a good conversation.

Should we want departures to be private affairs among old friends and family, or public affairs, a →generation drawing to its end, keeping company with each other?

SADNESS

Sadness comes and goes. During the Long Days, Last Months, and Last Weeks, there will be times that call for →laughter or a wry smile. You are not condemned to maintain a facade of sadness in honor of the seriously ill or as proof of your love of the Departing. Constant sadness may qualify as →depression. If someone at the bedside is resolutely tearful or intransigently grim, that person is in trouble.

Sadness comes in spurts, as the ill or Departing can no longer Drive
  Remember the day's events or exchanges {→Forgetfulness}
   Take a bath or shower unassisted
    Use the toilet unassisted
     Eat unassisted {→Food}
      Walk
       Sit on a commode
        Talk fluently
         Hold a book or magazine {→Reading}
         Breathe without →oxygen
         Swallow without difficulty
           Control bowels or urine, saliva or tears.
          Move the torso. The limbs.
         Move the head
          Speak or respond clearly
          Stay awake {→Sleep}

At each of these stages (which rarely proceed in this order, particularly for those previously disabled or disoriented), you may be further saddened by further losses of independence and expressions of selfhood. With each stage comes also a further loss of hope, further confirmation that the Departing is en route to departure.

The Departing may take this loss with more grace than you yourself can muster, a grace so moving that you are all the more deeply saddened. Or angered: how can a person of such grace be departing so soon under such grievous circumstances?

And then something truly funny will happen. When my father was no longer able to shape a coherent sentence or stay awake for more than a few minutes, my mother, brother, and I were in the living room with him watching *Jeopardy*. At one point during Alex Trebek's casual conversation with the contestants, Trebek asked for a show of hands in response to a question about their own experiences. Out of the blue my father raised his hand. He was, for the moment, still in the game.

SEASONS

More people commit (or succeed at) suicide in the spring than in any other season; the fewest commit (or succeed at) suicide in the winter. One would think it would be the opposite, and in fact more deaths worldwide occur in winter than during any other season. Deaths from stroke, from heart attacks and respiratory disorders, from diabetes and infectious diseases cluster in the winter. (Deaths from cancer or multiple sclerosis have no statistical correlation with any season.)

Global warming may lead to more summertime deaths than usual, from heatstroke, famine, drought, flooding, assault, and murder; if accompanied by more winter extremes, there will also be an exaggerated rate of winter mortality from respiratory illnesses, high winds, and, perhaps, from automobile accidents on icy roads.

SAD (Seasonal Affective Disorder) may play a role in lowering the resistance of people during months of least sun→light, so that those with terminal illnesses die of infections rather than directly of the illness, or simply lose the will to live. We have no statistics about the months, or temperatures, or humidities, during which people lose the will to live . . . or when we at the bedside become most impatient with the dying.

It is easier to sit at the bedside in the winter, when the world outside is most stormy, least seductive. And in the heat of the summer, when the coolness of a seat in a shaded room is preferable to the mean brilliance of the sun. Late spring and early fall would seem to be the most difficult of times, for then departure goes contrary to all the signs, the buds, the colors, the liveliness in the air, the first blossoms, the return to school after vacation.

Does →sitting at the bedside entail the sharing of gloom and discomfort, or an exchange of visions? Do we want the pathos of landscapes, where the inner and outer horizons mirror each other, or some humming, cranky contradiction, an outbreak of blessings?

Who chooses when to die by the rotation of the earth on its axis? Aren't there more important considerations?

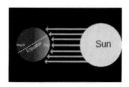

SELFISHNESS

Can it be selfish to want to live as long as humanly possible? Is clinging to life the last gasp of egoism when it means fatigue, frustration, and extended grief for all at the bedside? {→Buying Time, Readiness.} Is a drawn-out departure the ultimate narcissism? *I am dying, pay heed to me. My life. My passing*.

How disturbing to realize that you're entertaining such thoughts. It's blaming the victim, only worse. You may be at the end of your own rope, exhausted, out of tears and out of sorts, but you can't be in as bad a shape as the Departing. Die already!! you want to shout, but that would be inexcusable-- warrantable, maybe, but inexcusable. Time may be up {→ETD}, but the timing is up to the Departing, who seems willing to endure more →pain than ever you could, tolerate more physical losses than ever you would. If it were up to you, the →funeral would have taken place days ago: a kindness, for everyone.

But this is not a page about assisted suicide. {For some books and films on that: →Further Reading; Further Viewing.} This is a page about how those at bedsides begin to question the motives of those abed. Why is she still here? What more does he want of me? {→Anniversaries; Blackmail; *Quid Pro Quo.*} Is there something crucial he hasn't said? Something I haven't told her? Something yet to be done on behalf of a child or husband or niece or, who knows, the world? Does closure depend upon some last quest, or question answered? Why is all this anguish necessary?

Maybe it's not necessary. In addition to an instinct for survival, most of us have a repertoire of things we do *in extremis*, during the grimmest of moments: tactics for breathing under water. After decades of tragedies small and large, our recourse to these habits and tactics becomes automatic. Maybe that's what is happening now, and your job is to point this out, to assure the Departing that making do is no longer necessary. There are times when perseverance does not further.

Or maybe they are defiant. *I am not ready. You may be ready for my dying, but I need more time, more justice, more love. Who are you to suggest that I can't make do yet again?*

Such defiance may be an unreasonable, unseasonable assertion of an ongoing self in the face of implacable mortality. But isn't that what you do everyday upon rising: your yawn declares, Here I am. How selfless it would be for the Departing to depart without struggle, without asking for a minute more. A minute more.

SEX

Joyce, an intelligent woman who was also a quick reader of people and a ready wit, had been losing her short-term memory and her mobility. During her Last Days, in her eighties, she was confined to bed with pneumonia. Her husband at the bedside bent down to kiss her. She asked, "Does this mean we'll be having sex?"

The Departing do not forget about sex simply because they are preparing for departure. They may still want to look attractive, they may flirt in ways they have flirted since they were teens, and they often want more than a peck on the lips when a lover, wife, or husband bends down to kiss them. This may be shocking. Indeed, it may seem to those at the bedside almost necrophiliac, but the Departing (and the seriously ill) are not yet dead, not disembodied, and certainly not without desire {→Parking; Wives, Husbands, and Lovers.}

A regimen of opiates, or breakthrough →pain despite opiates, can so depress the libido that sex does not come into play. Similarly, →sadness and →fatigue can so depress the libido of those at the bedside that sex would appear to be the last thing on their agenda. And yet, one should not be surprised at how often intercourse, oral sex, or some sort of gentle sexplay or deeply sensuous massage is part of →hospice settings. Or can be, if you let it. {See also→Hands and Gloves.}

The ambition is rarely orgasm; it is closeness, the kind of embrace you want the night before you leave for a long tour of duty in a foreign country, or an open-ended road trip across continents. Sex as the finest companionship, the fullest love.

That sexual activity can happen during the Last Days does not mean that it must, or should. If it happens, it happens because it can happen. It is neither a final →signing off nor a last fling before a fall into the abyss. Don't make more of it than you make of the rest of the Last Weeks or Days. As it is not the End-All and Be-All of most lives beyond adolescence, it is not the End-All and Be-All of most deaths.

It is good, nonetheless. It can be very very good.

SHIT HAPPENS--OR NOT

Almost all analgesics cause constipation. Since most of the Departing are on powerful pain medications, they will be constipated, and they will complain about it.

They will almost invariably be on several kinds of laxatives:
1) lubricants that coat the bowels, and
2) softeners that soften the stools, both for easier passage;
3) hyperosmotics that draw water from tissues into the bowels,
4) and bulking agents that swell to form stools, both prompting peristaltic movements;
5) stimulants that increase contractions in bowel muscles that push the stool along.

After a while these all stop working, in part because the body is shutting down. The Departing, however, may still feel like having a bowel movement, or feel bloated because unable to have one, or feel upset about the distraction during a time that should be devoted to things more spiritual.

Although constipation can get in the way of "a good death" {→Deaths, Bad and Good}, it may also be a blessing, in that no one wants to be changing diapers or emptying a colostomy bag at the very end. Ideally, the body shuts down over several days, while the Departing drinks little and eats less, so that by the Last Hours there is no need to evacuate, no awkward sense of fullness. Ideally.

Often there will also be burping and flatulence. Flatus from fecal residues, or as a side-effect of laxatives, or from true constipation. This never happens in the movies. People on silver-screen deathbeds may be coughing up blood, but they never burp or fart{→Nothing Funny About This}.

How dare there be humor, scatological humor, in the Last Days! Dying is a serious business, with legal, financial, religious, and literary implications. Why then would anyone at the bedside pay attention to shit or piss or slow farts or a loud burp?

Because the body calls attention to itself, up to the last minute. It is the body, isn't it, that carries much of the burden of departure? So the body demands, and deserves, recognition. Our bodies, wasting away, becoming unhinged, still have more in common with each other than our cultures or local convenience stores. From birth, everyone shits, pisses, farts, burps, and screams. No shit, Sherlock: we are embodied creatures, our bodies with us to the end. We don't leave home without them, and none of us leaves for good without being reminded of them.

SHOES

Out of the blue it may hit you that the Departing has not put on shoes for a week or more. House slippers, perhaps, during the Last Months, then no shoes whatsoever. Of a sudden you know: the Departing will not be getting out of bed again, will no longer use that walker in the corner, that commode by the bedside, the support bar you installed in the shower. Will not be going outside.

This realization is often more heartbreaking than any medical prognosis. It is profoundly telling when the most humdrum of assumptions about how a person meets each day are no longer tenable.

In other societies, barefootedness may be less striking, but here in the West the shoes mean as much about possibility as about mobility. People put on their shoes to go out, meet other people, make things happen, remake themselves. The only people who die with their boots on are those who die →suddenly; the rest die stocking-footed or with bare feet.

You may have thought long and hard about what shoes to wear to the hospital or at the bedside {→Overnight Bags}. You know your shoes should be comfortable, because you will be there for a while, but should they be dressy, or basic, so you won't worry about any messes you may have to clean up? Who and what are the shoes representing, and who is going to care?

Respectability, empathy, resourcefulness, and independence come to be centered on shoes: "It's no use opening up an umbrella if your shoes leak"; "standing in someone else's shoes"; "cobbling together a life"; "if the shoe fits. . . ."

Which is why you may feel like a heel if you slip off your own shoes while at the bedside. Isn't that profoundly improper, demonstrating a lack of respect or a lackadaisical attitude toward your obligations to help with errands and sturdy support? Would taking off your shoes be a sign of settling in to be with the seriously ill over the long haul, or a sign that you are open to intimate conversation but not to the emptying of a urine collection bag?

At funerals with open caskets, morticians put shoes back on.

In the Days After, it may be more difficult to let go of the shoes of the Departing than of anything else in the closet. Well-worn shoes. Unworn shoes. Work shoes. Dress shoes. Shoes that no longer fit. Shoes that never did.

SIGNING OFF

Hints of impending departure may be observed through changes in metabolism and circulation that are not necessarily sudden but can appear so. As the →signs may seem to be contradictory, I list them here by contradictory pairs.

During the very Last Days, the Departing will:
sleep much and become difficult to wake;
become restless.
Even when awake and restless or making repetitive motions, the Departing may be unresponsive. This has nothing to do with you. The system is slowly shutting down. But there may be an hour of energized alertness shortly before departure.

experience difficulty swallowing and stop eating and drinking;
lick the lips.
Licking is a response to feelings of dry mouth or parched lips, not an appeal for food or water. Try glycerin swabs for lips, frozen juice chips for mouth or →tongue.

become pale or mottled and cooler to the touch;
sweat and kick off the covers.
A cool, or slightly warm, washcloth on the forehead may be a comfort; try both and look to see if the muscles of the face relax. Blankets may help forestall shivering.

make unusual requests of you, or recount specific visions;
become confused about time, place, and people in the room.
Be sure to identify yourself each time you talk to the Departing. Speak gently, in your own voice, not in a whisper or funereal tones. Honor requests that are simple and reasonable.

gurgle, or sound as if marbles were rolling around in the chest.
make fewer breathing sounds{Aspiration}
With less fluid intake, it's difficult to cough up normal secretions. It will help if the Departing turns her head to one side to aid drainage. His gurgling is not evidence of struggle, nor is a Cheyne-Stokes pattern of irregular shallow breaths with minute-long periods of no breathing whatever.

Very Important: Be sure to identify and contact beforehand the →physician who will be asked to sign the death certificate. Municipalities ordinarily require the signing to be done by a doctor who's seen the Departing within the last 2-3 weeks. If a →hospice is involved, this is easily taken care of; if hospice is not involved, this is very important, as often the Departing will not have seen a doctor recently.

SIGNS

What you may see at the bedside at each stage of departure:

Stage	~3 months	~1 month	~1-2 weeks	1-2 days
Alertness	inconsistent	sporadic; sleepy	mostly asleep	unresponsive
Anxiety	depression	restlessness	Agitation	little or none
Appetite	foods taste odd	soft foods only	liquids if at all	none
Blood pressure	slight decline	lower	lower yet	very low
Body temp	fever or sweating	alt. hot/cold	extremities cold	cold
Breathing	some wheezing or shallow breath	uneven, fast or slow, shallow	loud, irregular, puffing or stops	very irregular, rattling
Congestion	possible coughing	phlegm, mucous	aspiration	gurgling
Energy level	high, then low	low	low but surges	1 more surge?
Excretions	constip/diarrhea	slowing down	Minimal	final loosening
Mental acuity	forgetfulness, inattentiveness	confusion, loss of focus	Often oblivious strange dreams	momentary
Mobility	muscle weakness, dizziness	hard to walk – bed-ridden	cannot stand, hard to sit up	none
Phys. dexterity	slow decline	hard to feed self	very little	none
Pulse/heart rate	Uneven	extremes:40-150	150 down to 0	approaching 0
Skin	much sweating	bedsores, dryness	itchy, blotchy	yellowing
Smell (sense of)	little change	peculiar intolerances	extreme in- or high sensitivity	none to speak of
Sociability	alt. withdrawal/ engagement	intermittent and short-term	decreasing	little or none
Speech	some slowness	circular, failing	phrases only	single words
Thirst	increased	dry mouth	Declining	none
Throat	sensitive	hard to swallow	painful	gurgling
Time (sense of)	shortened/tense	haphazard	Floating	tenuous
Touch (sense of)	acute	damped	Dulled	dull
Vision	some faintness peripheral loss	hallucinations sleep	some cloudiness much sleep	looking inward eyes glassy

Warning! Do not read this chart as fateful. If you observe many of the signs in, say, column 2, by no means assume that death is inevitable within a month {→ETD} People do rebound, even when presenting with the signs in column 4, particularly when a serious illness turns out to have been the result of wrongly prescribed or mismanaged drugs, to allergic reactions, to poor wound care, or to surgical error {→Iatrogenesis}. Moreover, no two people follow identical or smooth trajectories toward recovery or departure.

SITTING

As in childcare.
As in toilet training.
As in →waiting.
As in keeping company.
As in meditation.
As in "sit down, I need to tell you something."
As in taking an exam.
As in non-violent protest.
As in mourning.

During the Last Months you will sit. For hours. Sitting for hours, you will be reminded of other times you sat for hours, waiting for someone to get out of surgery, for a car to be repaired, a form to be processed. Each of those other stints of sitting seems to have prepared you for this, particularly when the person abed is fitfully asleep or knocked out.

Sitting demands discipline. Buddhist sitting is about being fully present to a world ever in flux. Jewish sitting (or *shiva*, or *sheva*) is about mourning for seven days in the presence of your community, each of whose members has a memory to share of the Departing or a secret that must now be revealed.

Sitting may feel like an utmost futility, the opposite of *doing*, but in the Last Days sitting at the bedside is *doing*, and hard to do. Because you want to get away. Because you are restless about your own life. Because you need to stretch your legs.

So, stretch your legs, often.
→Read to the Departing, even if she appears to be asleep.
Sing {→Music}.
Hold →hands with the Departing, though unconscious.
Talk quietly, even to yourself.

How else do you sit for hours?

You stretch your legs.
You massage your legs, especially the calves {→Cramping}.
You recollect.
You make lists of things to do, people to call {→Checklists}
You drift off {→Generations}

The Departing drifts off, does not return.

You rise.

SKILLED NURSING FACILITIES (SNFs)

Pronounced "sniffs," SNFs are transitional between hospital and home. At least, this is Medicare's notion: it will cover up to 100 days of acute care in a SNF, *per illness*, within 30 days after a person has been in hospital for that illness three consecutive nights. The 30-days provision means that hospital patients who need continuing care can opt for discharge back →home, to see whether they can get along with a visiting nurse before deciding to enter a SNF. Medicare pays for →nursing visits at home 2-3 times/week; it covers SNF costs for the first 20 days, including ambulance from hospital to SNF, then requires a co-pay for the next 80,* coverable through some Medigap policies.

→"Acute care" is care through which a person is likely to improve, as assessed by SNF staff who review the progress of patients each week. When no further improvement is seen or foreseen, a patient must be discharged home or to a facility that attends to those who need help with activities of daily living (ADLs) such as toileting, bathing, dressing. Pursuant to a recent court decision, however, Medicare may now cover care in a SNF for those unlikely to improve but in need of significant daily nursing care so as to maintain their current viable status.

I focus on Medicare because the majority of admissions to SNFs arrive under its aegis. Private insurance plans for those not (yet) eligible for Medicare have similar provisos. Long-term health insurance may pay for non-medical help at a board and care and should pay for care in a SNF beyond the first 100 days.

At a board-and-care, unlike a SNF, staff may empty catheter bags but may not flush or change →catheters or give injections. Hospice-certified board-and-cares can help with →oxygen.

To confuse matters, SNFs often have wings dedicated to custodial care, coinciding with the older notion of retirement homes, which are basically board-and-cares. If a SNF has separate units, one of which provides close medical supervision with RNs available 24-7, it is akin to multi-stage Assisted Living facilities that provide meals, maid service, and transport for the more independent. An Assisted Living facility may include a separate "memory care" unit for those with Alzheimer's. A new type of care facility is also emerging: patient-centered medical homes: www.vtafp.net/vtafp/PCMH Template.pdf.

*It's actually more complicated: www.medicare.gov/Pubs/pdf/10050.pdf

SLEEP

The seriously ill and Departing may sleep so deeply that you become troubled, alarmed. Did you exhaust her with your questions and →checklists? Is he avoiding the family? Is she escaping the racket made by her roommate in this facility? Is he trying to elude a →Bounty Hunter? Did she overdo the fentanyl lollipop? Is she going into a full-fledged coma?

Relax, and get some sleep yourself. You need a good nap, and better a full night's sleep. If you worry so much about peaceful sleeping, what state will you be in nearer the end?

Agreed, the sleep of the seriously ill and Departing is not always peaceful (though nightmares are rare unless there has been an opiate overdose). They may be muttering or calling out, twitching and →turning. And the breathing pattern can be distressingly uneven, with periods as long as minutes during which there is no breath going in or out, and then, whammo! spurts of fast breathing. This is not because they are dreaming of running sprint relays. It may be sleep apnea, which is likely to have been a problem for years, but during the Last Days it's also how the lungs and metabolism approach death.

Do not force pills on anyone while asleep for long periods; do not try to feed solid foods. Pudding or applesauce may be ok (the Departing can swallow semi-automatically), but feeding is not critical. Apply glycerin to the lips so that they do not crack. Slide a pillow under the legs so that the ankles and heels are not rubbing against the mattress or each other, to prevent →bedsores. That's about it.

A day later, or three, they will wake up feeling refreshed, with things on their minds, as if they had been making lists while sleeping, or feeling chatty, as if words had earned a reprieve. They will not apologize for the long sleep nor be concerned about what day it is; when you tell them, they will be mildly interested, especially if it is the Sabbath.

A few hours later, the cycle is likely to repeat: long deep sleep; waking in a generally good mood, probably →thirsty, possibly hungry {→Food}. Until the cycle no longer repeats.

If you expected the Last Days to be filled with conversation, reminiscence, and mutual admissions, you are going to be disappointed by the long deep sleeps. If you expected writhing, anguish, and terror, you will be relieved. If you allow yourself to relax into this cycle, you too may be refreshed when the Departing wakes. And when, at last, there is only sleep, you may be→sad but not frantic.

SOCIAL WORKERS

Although social workers seem frequently to appear out of the blue, they are not miracle workers. Whether as hospital discharge planners, nursing home ombudspersons, assisted living supervisors, or explicitly as social workers for county agencies, they mean to help, and they can. They know about →caretaking and →respite options. They can arrange for assistance with medical-financial issues. They can coordinate efforts with bureaucracies and serve as liaisons between medical and social services. They can help you find home health aides, housekeepers, or companions. They can unknot institutional double binds. They can listen to family and friends and sketch out a comprehensive support system. They can put you in touch with counselors and →bereavement groups.

Social workers can also intrude. County, state, and federal laws require them to report circumstances that you might prefer to go unreported. Despite (or because of) their training, they can be moralistic and judgmental. They may apply their own criteria to →quality-of-life decisions already made.

One historian has called them "professional altruists." Trained to act on behalf of others, they assume that they will always have at heart their best interests. As professionals, they pride themselves on being objective altruists; that is, they may believe that they can see what the seriously ill and Departing need far better than close friends and family whose vision is clouded by affection, grief, or lifelong patterns of craziness.

It is good to get the perspective of social workers, and to get access through them to federal, state, county, and local agencies. During the Last Days, however, professional altruism is not what is needed. There can be many reasons why you are at the bedside: indebtedness; love; reciprocation; habit; greed; friendship; protectiveness; guilt; a desire for reconciliation; financial or occupational circumstances that make it easier for you to be there than others; the sharing of the experience of an illness that, in your case, has turned out not to be terminal, not yet terminal. Whatever the reasons (ordinarily plural), your presence at the bedside is neither professional nor entirely altruistic.

Which is as it must be. There are no pure motives for tending to a sick or dying person, and it is helpful to realize that, for your own sake. It is too great a burden on all concerned during the Long Days, Last Months, Weeks, or Days to carry oneself as if a saint who seems too good to be true, too sweet to be kind, too helpful to be of help.

SPEECH

So much to say, so much to tell, so many questions to ask, yet here you are at the bedside and there's no hint of conversation The person in the bed is asleep most of the time, or on pain meds and unresponsive, or defiantly taciturn.

You could understand it if there were aphasia, a neurological deficit in the speech centers of the brain, caused by stroke, brain injury, or meningitis. If speech were impaired but recoverable, you would have a role: helping with exercises set up by speech pathologists; tracking the degree of recovery.

You could understand it if there were speech problems due to a feeding →tube, or to medical-mechanical problems with poor dentition, burns affecting the tissues of the →throat. You could contrive non-verbal languages--alphabet boards for pointing out individual letters and numbers; a white board on which to make and erase marks; a code of winks, nods, sniffs, pinches.

And although it would be hard, you could still understand it if all language were confused, incoherent, unintelligible or drably repetitive due to senility, dementia, Alzheimer's, or whatever it's being called this month. Some people, like those with Parkinson's, can sing fluently when they can no longer speak.

You could even understand it, maybe, if there were muteness from severe shock or loss, or from a multitude of indeterminate causes, so long as the doctors were talking with you about what they had in mind to do about it, and what you might do.

But when the silence can be imputed to your own presence? Maybe you are missing a subtle attempt at communication, →eyes beseeching you, a finger curling, a tongue pressed momentarily against a bottom lip.

We are speaking animals. Animals that speak more than words: we have grammar, syntax, inflection, and through them we shape our worlds with figures of speech, simile and metaphor. Our history is words. So now what?

You stay for a while.
Sometimes you hum: could this prompt a soundful exchange?
Or you bring in some →music that he always loved, listening for what happens.
Or you talk with others at the bedside, in calm tones; maybe she will join in, or moan to tell you to knock it off.

During the Long Days, there will usually come a time for words. In the Last Days, no promises. In either case, it's not up to you. Really.

STAGES

1969. After working with terminally ill patients in hospitals and clinical practice, the psychiatrist Elizabeth Kübler-Ross published her seminal work, *On Death and Dying*, which laid out the five stages of loss or grief through which the Departing go as they come to terms with their dying:

Denial and isolation ("This can't be happening. Go away.")
Anger and blame ("I won't stand for this. Who did this to me?)
Bargaining ("If I can live to see X or do Y, I'll go peacefully.")
Depression ("   ")
Acceptance ("OK everyone, it's time.")

These are often taken to be necessary stages. They are better understood as angles of response, openings for insight. Bereavement counselors may go so far as to track the grief of those at the bedside by Kübler-Ross stages, with cautions not to skip a stage or skip too quickly ahead. Not to follow the protocol would of course set one back--to the first stage, Denial.

Still and all, the stages through which the Departing are supposed to go may not be the same as the stages you go through at the bedside. Sticking with fives, we might expect something like an economic sequence for those at the bedside:

Gathering ("Tell me again, I don't quite understand.")
Hunting & Fishing ("There must be something else to try.")
Farming ("We need supplies for tending to this dying person.")
Manufacturing ("What must I prepare for now? And now?)
Service Industries ("I am here for you.")

Sixes make more emotional sense, and form a backwards acronym: DURESS.

Shock ("I wasn't prepared for it to come so soon.")
Seeking Second Opinions ("Is it really a death sentence?")
Emptiness & Meditation ("What can I possibly say? I don't have my own life figured out, yet here I am.")
Relenting & Redefining ("OK, how can I help now that the end is so near?")
Useful Mediation ("What does the Departing need of me? What do I want from him/her?")
Disengagement ("I know, I know, I have to let go, there's no point in prolonging the departure, it's selfish to think that death waits upon me.")

If we add a seventh stage, the acronym becomes: ASSURED: Acknowledgment. ("I am grateful for, indebted to...")
Acknowledgments never lay blame.

STRENGTH

Strength of character, strength of purpose, strength of mind, strength of love . . . strength, strength, strength, strength. Eight letters with only one vowel, the short *e* distributing its energy among all the consonants, holding them together.

You never ask the ill or Departing to "buck up" or "take it like a man." {→Women and Men} They may be stoic, but you don't ask them for stoicism, which rather isolates than affirms.

Some try to hold everything together during the Last Days; others take the Last Days as an invitation to abandon the pretence. By definition, the Departing can't be as strong as once they once were, can't be the sustaining force in a family, a couple, a network of friends, or a way of life.

The Departing, however, may believe that strength is required of them until their final breaths. They may believe that they need to be wholly present for whoever is at the bedside, a presence that demands of them a strength they have rarely summoned before. They are being strong for you.

Or they believe that departure becomes indecent where they are utterly dependent on nurses and caregivers, or under the tug of narcotics. So they hang in there, asserting as much of themselves as is left to assert, straining to be decent, to make no disgraceful spectacle of themselves as one system after another fails and they succumb.

What an odd word, "succumb." Seven letters and two *u*'s, or you's. Succumbing is a gerund of relationship: you succumb to something, someone. You do not so much yield as lose the capacity to defy. You do not construct the terms of surrender; you succumb.

In that absence of resistance and a gradual or sudden loss of self-definition {→Identity}, the weakness of the Departing becomes most patent and painful. There and then you tell yourself, now *I* must be strong.

Strong for what? Strong for whom? Those are not rhetorical questions. At the bedside of a once-purposive person, you must reflect, and answer. What is that *e* doing? What are the *e*-ssentials in strength?

You may have convinced yourself that staying strong is better than breaking down, going haywire, and drawing attention away from the Departing, as if jealous of the macabre spotlight. That's probably true, but it's half an answer, the easy half. Strong for what? Strong for whom?

SUDDENNESS

Everyone has been waiting for it for days, weeks, months, yet when the departure occurs, it can seem sudden. Why?

Because, no matter what anyone tells you, there's no intermediate stage between breathing and not breathing. (I'm asthmatic; I know.)

Because, dying is not the same as being dead.

Because hopelessness is impossible among the living. To be entirely hopeless is not to take another breath.

Because each departure proceeds at a different rhythm, and no one can be relied upon to give you solid estimates of the final hour, half hour {→Cascades, ETD}.

Because there's always something you've put off, something you've been meaning to say or ask, and just as the Departing is departing you'll remember what it was.

Because few ever announce: Now I'm going to die. {→Last Breaths}.

Because the Departing often choose to depart in your absence.

Because time slows at the bedside but at the departure it speeds up. A whirlwind of activity follows: calls, e-mails, texts, appointments, errands. And the world impinges {→Checklists; Funeral Arrangements; Obituaries}.

Because rentals (beds, air mattresses, →oxygen pumps) are swiftly removed and geographies change: you're no longer in the same place each day, or the space is...emptier. In this sense, a departure can seem like moving day.

Because there's just so much steeling against death that anyone can do.

Even you.

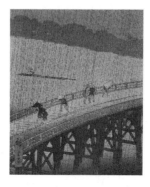

TEETH

Decay: civilizations; monuments; morals; manners; teeth. Always an afterthought, tooth decay is often neglected during the Long Days and →Last Months.

O say it is not so.

For dental health is related to general fortitude, dental decline to other immediate and systemic problems.

Toothache, certainly, can be blindingly painful, and must be dealt with quickly, particularly where a nerve is exposed. But even in the absence of pain and oral hypersensitivity, tooth decay and gum diseases may have stern consequences.

People with periodontal disease are almost twice as likely to have coronary artery disease, and a high incidence of gingivitis or cavities is as good a predictor of heart disease as high levels of cholesterol. A similarly startling statistical relationship holds between periodontal disease and stroke: Dr. Moise Desvarieux of Columbia University has shown that those with high levels of certain disease-causing bacteria in the mouth are more likely to have atherosclerosis in the carotid artery in the neck, which can lead to stroke. In addition, studies of the bacteria in plaque and in oral biofilms (bacterial and fungal pathogens that form a nearly invisible slime) reveal that their proliferation may lead to infections around the heart. Finally, periodontal bacteria entering the bloodstream can hamper the body's ability to control insulin levels among those with diabetes.

Vice versa, systemic disorders such as Crohn's disease may be at the root of a progressive inflammation of the gums. Oral infections by fungi and herpes are common in those with impaired immunity or autoimmune disorders, such as patients with (and receiving chemotherapy for) cancer or AIDS.

Further, there are causal relationships among temporo-mandibular joint (TMJ) problems, tooth malformations, and the occurrence of migraines or hearing loss.

SO, aside from the obvious benefits of eliminating mouth odor, improving mouthfeel, and avoiding toothache, those at the bedside should encourage dental hygiene and professional cleanings. An alcohol-free mouthwash after each meal, with flossing, will work better than an incomplete or inept brushing morning and night. Mobile dentists can come to the bedside to conduct inspections and perform cleanings.

Should I have subtitled this chapter "a brush with death"?

"THINGS HAPPEN FOR A REASON."

They do not.

Or they do, but each person at the bedside has in mind a different reason.

Or they do, but no one is sure of the reason, whether informed by predestination, divine purpose, karma, fate, or chaos theory.

People say "Things happen for a reason" not because they have figured out the reason but because they think it will be comforting for all to know that this illness or departure, like every other illness or departure, cannot be random or plain unlucky. {Consider→Accidentals; Ethical Wills; Have You Thought Of...}

Whether or not things happen for a reason, saying that they do is cold comfort during a long excruciating illness or in the Last Days. Either you know the reason or you don't. If you are certain of the reason, then you may be inveigled into blaming someone, something. A reason is never so innocent as to forestall regret and recrimination. If you don't know the reason, or if the reasons are disputed, then you will spend more time dissecting the past (a reason is always in the past) than seeing to the present, and you risk disturbing whatever calm has been managed.

What happens during the Last Days has its own logic, its own rhythm and progression, and proceeds determinedly enough without a reason.

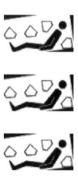

THIRST

Not eating is easier to take lightly than not drinking. How many times have you heard that no one can live more than three days without water? In emergency rooms, don't they presume that most people are dehydrated and need IV fluids?

During the Last Weeks, the Departing gradually lose their ability to swallow and their desire to eat. For a while longer, less because they are thirsty than because their mouths feel annoyingly dry, or because the mucous in their throats is salty, they will continue to sip fluids when offered (water, thin juices, Gatoraid, iced tea) or willingly suck on ice chips. Then, during the Last Days or Last Hours, they will not drink anything.

In hospital, physicians or nurses will remove the IV →tubes and bags of fluid that have ordinarily been in place to keep the person hydrated. These fluids are of two kinds, crystalloid or colloidal, depending on the kind of fluid balance needed. Crystalloids such as saline or Ringers LR solution promote electrolyte replacement but have become controversial because they are pro-inflammatory; dextrose protects against cellular dehydration but may be contraindicated for those with very low blood pressure. Colloids such as albumin, mannitol, or dextran improve fluid volume but also increase edema. (Read Kim David, RN, "IV fluids: Do you know what's hanging and why" in www.modernmedicine.com [October 1, 2007].)

When the Departing stops wanting to drink and refuses liquids, departure will occur within the week {→Signs}.

This can be hard to take. Physically hard {→Preparing the Body}. It's impossible not to empathize with someone whose →throat is parched. Dry. Parched.

You, however, must drink. Like mothers who tend to hold their breath in sympathy with a child having an asthma attack, those at the bedside may--without realizing it--try to keep such close company with the Departing as to go without food and water.

Stumbling, dizziness, edginess: if someone at the bedside has these symptoms, or a peculiar inattentiveness or atypical awkwardness, bring a large glass of juice or water and insist that it be downed immediately, slowly, and entirely. (Not a soda, not coffee, not a shake. Just juice or water.) Accept no delays or equivocations. Dehydration leads to constipation, which leads to irritableness, which leads in turn to impatience and bad decisions. Serious dehydration leads directly to the emergency room. . . .Think of drinking at the bedside as a toast to the Departing.

TONGUES

Trust naturopaths and ayurvedic healers on this: the tongue shows more than it tells.

Aside from noting the creamy white lesions of thrush (*candida*) and the danger of epileptics "swallowing" their tongues during seizures, Western doctors tend to let the tongue slide in their examinations and diagnoses, while healers across the world consider the state(ments) of the tongue more intently. Is it fuzzy? Furrowed? Is it green, blue, purple, yellow? Does it seem to droop, loll, or curl up?

Critical as the tongue is to →speech and singing, to lovemaking and winetasting, why is it so overlooked by modern medicine? Why do we have at hand age-old tongue depressors, to get the tongue out of the way, but no tongue assessors? As adults we have learned the signs of colds, flu, allergies, measles, mumps, but do you know what it means when a tongue has become black and hairy? Or "geographic," pocked with reddish shapes that resemble land masses on a relief map? (Geographic Tongue is actually "benign migratory glossitis," or so says medicinenet, at www.medicinenet.com.)

Check the standard medical sources and you will find that nearly every odd appearance of the tongue is dismissed as benign, cosmetic, or peripheral to something more serious such as scarlet fever.

In naturopathy, as in non-Western medicine, the status of the tongue is significant. It is no mere outlier (out-liar?) but an index to the caliber of nutrition, the onset of a disease, the progress of a therapy. It may expose subtle reactions to environmental toxins, florid reactions to prescription drugs. This is not the place for a manual of tongue diagnostics, but I bring up the tongue because you too, helping feed someone, or fetching toothpaste, or bending close to make out a few words, will notice changes in the texture, color, and topography of the tongue. And you too may wonder why no nurse or doctor is more directly addressing the tongue.

Is it because the tongue forked or slanderous is associated with deception, and one cannot trust it either to speak or show truth? Or because it is so forceful a causal agent in →politics, investing, and marketing that modern medicine is reluctant to allow the tongue any similar prerogative in the human body, its own scientific precinct? Or because the tongue entices, seduces, and must be resisted as Odysseus resisted the Sirens, who were really no more than animals?

Balderdash. Swill. Codswallop. Twaddle.

TRIAGE

Triage, or a system of assigning priorities of medical care, may begin long before an emergency room and continue long after.

Triage is already in effect, socioeconomically, with regard to who receives (or does not receive) preventive care and who has immediate (or delayed, or no) access to fine clinics, specialists, private beds, private duty nurses,→case managers.

Triage is already in effect, sociomedically, with regard to who rises (or does not rise) to the top of national lists for a liver or kidney transplant, or a new heart {→Organ Donation}.

Triage is already in effect, sociolegally, with regard to the implementation of end-of-life preferences {→DNR; Wills}.

Triage is already in effect in the drug formularies of insurance companies, who may refuse to pay for experimental drugs that have had no better success than a placebo.

Here I must digress. The placebo effect is not something to sneer at. If I am pain-free for hours in a dentist's chair after taking a pill presented as a new analgesic, why would I be upset to find out it's sugarpaste? "I shall please," says the placebo, and it does, so long as I don't know it's a placebo. The problem is that we assume that if something can be remedied using a placebo, it's not real or serious. Since a placebo relies on trust and works upon beliefs, it must be effective when the pain or illness is only in the mind. But what does it mean to be "only in the mind," given that the brain has a major role in producing sensations of pleasure and pain throughout the body? (The vagus nerve, I should note, is also implicated in producing or sustaining placebo effects.)

The reasoning that leads to a dismissiveness of placeboes affects triage in the ER, hospital, and →SNF. Nurses and orderlies defer helping people whose problems are "only in the mind," and move on to cases of profuse bleeding, gasping for breath, facial paralysis. Unlike daily triage among children and parents, medical triage does not sequence care according to the duration of screaming or the degree of pain visible on a face, since pain and its expressions are subjective--"in the mind."

Sitting at the bedside of someone who is shrieking, you will become furious when it takes eighteen minutes for a hospital or SNF nurse to show up with more painkiller. It's clearly not how you would respond at the bedside at home, where pain relief can be paramount. Triage is a term for dealing with populations, not with a person.

TUBES

Leading up to the end is a wild kelp garden of tubes: IV tubes into the arms, →oxygen tubes into the nose, →catheters and superpubic tubes, ostomy tubes, feeding tubes, breathing tubes, morphine pumps, all intertwined with the wires of heart monitors, telephones, call buttons, pressure cuffs on the legs to ward off blood clots.

One thrashing nightmare and all the tubes and wires can become a second nightmare, almost hilarious. Almost {→Nothing Funny About This}.

During the Last Days, the tubes disappear, one by one, two by two. It is a frightening liberation.

As the tubes are removed, the Departing is freed for departure and looks more human, but those tubes were also sustaining *you*, weren't they? They were lifelines between you, the Departing, and the doctors and nurses who know how to keep people breathing and aware. The tubes were also lifelines to the powered world beyond, to the dynamos, hydroelectric dams, wind turbines, oil derricks and refineries that make all this electricity and tubing possible: civilization at its most desperately redemptive.

As a person seems to shrink, tubes and wires compensate for the shrinkage, extending the body into four full dimensions, arcing into strangely beautiful tangents, translucent, green, yellow, blue. When the tubes and leads and wires vanish, it's already something of a death, a premonition of the incorporeal {→Diminishing}.

So you may be taken aback by, and even dispute, the removal of tubes, when in fact during the Last Days you should be an active →advocate for their removal, especially those tubes connected to in-room monitors so impatiently sensitive that they buzz and beep for no good reason throughout the day and →night, disturbing everyone.

In the medieval Everyman plays, our bodies are called "bags of bones." Once plastics and copper filaments and rubber insulation came along, we found that we were a tent and tempest of tubules.

When the tubes outside vanish and the tubules inside burst or disintegrate, there is nothing left but to go home.

TURNING

Four or five times each night, each of us goes through a cycle from shallow →sleep (Stage I) to very deep sleep (Stage IV). During Stages III and IV, we toss and turn until we lie entirely still for a period of Stage IV called REM--rapid eye movement--sleep. Most of our dreams occur during this REM period.

REM is the kind of sleep from which it is most difficult to wake; if a clock-radio screams us out of REM sleep, we wake shaken. Everyone at the bedside needs not only to get enough sleep but to get enough REM sleep, for in addition to sleep deprivation there is such a thing as dream deprivation. Sleeping pills and many kinds of anti-depressants can suppress dreaming. Dream loss, in turn, can make people clinically →depressed.

The Departing also dream, inside and outside of REM sleep; during sleep Stages III and IV they toss and turn much less than the rest of us. A modicum of tossing and turning is good for the body; otherwise the skin is susceptible to →bedsores.

One of the sadder →signs of the Last Months or weeks is when the Departing no longer toss and turn in their sleep and can no longer turn themselves in bed while awake. You must help them turn every few hours so as to avoid bedsores, cramps, sore muscles. They do not have to be turned much, just three or four inches to the left or the right, with pillows assuring that pressure is shifted.

But how do you turn someone who is "dead weight," and possibly heavier than you are? Beneath the torso should be a draw sheet (or "pull sheet") that runs across the center of the bed. If you roll-and-fold the draw sheet on one side until it is up against the body of the Departing, then pull straight on that roll-fold as if trying to pull the sheet out from under the Departing, s/he will begin to turn to the other side, and you can place a pillow as a brace in the space cleared. DO NOT pull up, because then you will be trying to lift the full weight; instead, pull flat along the mattress surface. If there is no draw sheet, the same technique can be used with a regular sheet, but because of its lengthwise extent, you will need help.

→Nurses and home health aides know how to do this. Watch them, or ask for a demonstration. At home you may need to turn the bedridden every two or three hours, but you may not need to wake in the middle of the night to turn them unless they have early signs of bedsores.

After all, you need to do yourself a good turn and get your own sleep, your own dreams.

UGLINESS

Bad taste haunts the bedside: in hospitals and nursing homes, art so inoffensive it can but offend the connoisseur's eye; at hospice or at home, commercial bouquets so badly arranged that no florist would claim credit; in the mail, cards so treacly that the sentiments behind them become instantly suspect.

And however you might wish that a person could be arranged in bed in some artful way, in some visually restful position, with soothing →music on a soulful soundtrack, there will be ugly times that violate every aesthetic principle: gross incontinence, →bleeding, bruising from badly-situated IVs, the guggle of mucous and saliva. You are wise enough not to blame him for interrupting your idyll, kind enough not to reprimand her for awful sounds and unpleasant →odors, but you think to yourself, "If I were writing this script, it would so much better for everyone"--dying as Easy Listening.

I exaggerate. No one could have such bad taste as to judge a departure by its clean lines, could they? No one would judge the Departing by the rumple of bed linens or tangle of tubing. But this is not to say we wouldn't want it otherwise, all things being equal.

Is it in bad taste to look for the dying to be characteristic of the living, confluent with the person we believe we know. We want, sometimes desperately, to understand the style and tempo of a departure as the culminating expression of the life of the Departing. {See also →Anniversaries, Cascades, Readiness.} Why shouldn't the Last Months and Days be arranged as a final, coherent act?

Oh, we know we shouldn't expect and can't demand such coherence, and it would be in the worst taste to ask the Departing to play a more fetching or graceful part in the departure, and yet----

Who just brought in that abominable vase?

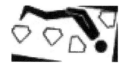

UPSTAIRS

"Sick rooms" used to be put at the top of a house, away from commotion and the →odors of outhouses or indoor plumbing. That was in the era of servants, call bells, and kitchens with dumbwaiters. (Only for the well-off, to be sure.)

Today the ideal is to have the seriously ill on the same floor as the kitchen, a toilet, and a step-in shower. Their rooms should be well ventilated and easily heated. From their beds they should have clear views out a →picture window and toward a tv screen. No stairs or steps should impede or endanger mobility.

This ideal benefits the sick, their guests, and their →caregivers. Stairs are almost as great a handicap to principal caregivers as for those in wheelchairs or prone to →falling. Caregivers themselves may already have bad knees, lung problems, or arthritis; if not careful, they may develop lower back problems.

Elevators are good things, especially in apartment buildings, but few private homes have them and most families cannot afford them. Installed inside, they cost $25-30,000; as an external add-on with its own foundation, at least $40,000. New "vacuum elevators" fit into smaller indoor spaces; they can cost as little as $20,000.

Electromechanical stair chairs/lifts are cheaper (~$2000 for a single flight, including installation; more if the chair must go around a bend or across a landing up a second flight). Such lifts are useful for those who can walk on the flat but not upstairs, and for those in wheelchairs who can transfer easily. Because the lifts are slow, they are of little help in urgent (toileting or medical) situations and caregivers themselves almost never use them.

Always a concern of →case managers working toward the discharge of patients from hospitals is the physical layout at home. Stairs, whether at the entry or up to a bath or bedroom or toilet, may be a deterrent to discharge back home, entailing a stay at a →SNF or board-and-care until the layout is changed, since recuperation depends on patient safety and caregiver energy, both of which can be compromised by stair-climbing. Entryway ramps may need to be built, a bed moved onto the same floor as toilet and bath, a bathtub or shower revamped. When a person lives in a second- or third-story walk-up, a new residence may have to be found.

Peculiar, how the emotional terrain of a disease or injury bears an inverse relation to the topography of one's living space.

URGENCY

So friends & relatives fly in from all over the globe & there are instructions on the bureau & the bedtable & bathroom mirror & refrigerator about what to do in case of this or that & everyone says there isn't much time left, it could happen at any moment, & everyone needs to be brought up to speed on what's been happening, what's likely to happen, what's sure to happen, and you're telling them all, one after the other, & it's so dizzying you're out of breath from the hushed talking or the travel or the loss of sleep or the anticipation or no exercise for days & a bad diet but there's so much to be done, papers to be sorted, arrangements to be made & confirmed, calls & messages to return, prescriptions to fill, more calls to return, & that's why you're here, isn't it, to be helpful, to make known your concern and affection for the Departing in this final time of need, or for the family of the Departing, & you're trying to remember that note to yourself you'd made mentally but forgot to write down yesterday when you should have, it seemed so important at the time.

Calm down people keep telling you & you're calm enough at the bedside. In fact, it's something of a relief to take your place at the bedside, because then you can fall into another rhythm, rather of slow release than of flap&flurry. There you can keep time with the Departing, although in the back of your mind you're still a little worried about what you'll need to do for breakthrough →pain or vomiting . . .

This business of busyness at the bedside comes of the awkwardness of the Last Days, which are inevitably slipped into the middle of other ongoing days for so many other ongoing people. Treat the Last Days as an ultimatum, a deadline one rushes to meet, and you meet up more often than not with the resistance of the Departing themselves. Treat the Last Days as the collapse of time, when hours and minutes are relative only to the amount of pain the Departing is in, and you begin to fear that you are losing your own footing in the world. Treat the Last Days as a continuing crisis, and you work yourself into a blizzard of →checklists.

The true urgency of a departure lies in whatever fear, joy, love, or gratefulness remains to be expressed between you and the Departing. Aside from violating a →DNR, no serious mistakes can be made during the →Last Days so long as you are quietly attentive while at the bedside. Attentiveness need not be busyness, and busyness can mask inattentiveness. Next page. Now.

URGENCY, AGAIN

What the Departing needs from you is neither the shrill alarm of a clockwinder nor the deep calm of a spiritual master but the responsiveness of a good ear and warm→hand. That you feel →anxious, distressed, or strangely distant is not unusual or inappropriate. To be more preoccupied with the furious details of an impending death than is the Departing, that can be a problem, for then your sense of time will not be in accord with the Departing's sense of time. In consequence, it will be hard to agree on what is mutually important to do in the remaining hours.

Speed does not →buy more time. It is important to be quick in the relief of pain, but fluster and flutter at the bedside actually amplify pain, for wild urgency exaggerates *your* situation, *your* anxiety, and even the Departing struggle toward empathy for as long as needs be.

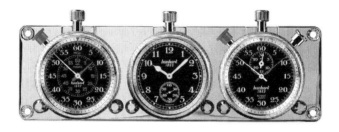

VETERANS

Seven per cent of Americans, some 22,000,000 men and women, are military veterans. Of these, 9,000,000 are sixty-five or over, and that number will grow. Each year, 500,000 veterans go through their Last Days; each week, 10,000 die.

When reaching their Last Months, veterans often enter Veterans Hospitals, which have their own end-of-life nursing staff if not also a →hospice team.

On pensions at death, see {→Death Benefits} and also www.dva.gov.au/pensions/yandyp/frontpg.htm. Chapter 8, What To Do When Someone Dies, is particularly helpful.

Upon request, the VA furnishes at no charge a headstone or marker for the grave of any deceased veteran in any cemetery around the world. Benefits may also include a gravesite in any of 125 national cemeteries that have space available, as well as opening and closing of the grave, a burial flag, and perpetual care. Similar benefits may extend to a veteran's spouse, to children under eighteen, and to adult dependents. Some are eligible for Burial Allowances. Speak with a Veterans benefits counselor at 1-800-827-1000. Don't wait on this: →paperwork can be time-consuming.

In general, burial benefits extend to:
--any member of the Armed Forces who dies on active duty;
--anyone who was honorably discharged from service after 9/7/80 (enlisted person) or 10/16/81 (officer) and served a full tour of duty;
--any U.S. citizen whose "last active service was terminated honorably";
--the spouse of an eligible veteran,
--certain dependents.
There are also provisions with regard to memorializing soldiers missing in action.

I quote, condense, or paraphrase most of this directly from the VA website, www.vba.va.gov/survivors/index.htm. Check this for updates and changes.

P.S. "Honor Flights" for a one-day visit to the war monuments and the Air & Space Museum in Washington, D.C., are now being offered, free of charge, to all veterans of World War II. These flights, which take off once or twice a month from many different cities, are staffed by physicians, nurses, and a host of volunteers to help veterans who are disabled, on oxygen, or otherwise fragile For more information: www.honorflight.org.

VOMIT

With certain cancers and liver disease, vomiting is inevitable. Iin the Last Months it is a near-certainty. The vomiting comes of a system that is slowing down and can no longer process what it once processed effortlessly; it comes of a reaction to deep pain or to medications that relieve pain; it comes from problems with swallowing or from the →anxiety that follows an episode of choking.

Emesis, the technical term, does not make vomiting any more pleasant, and those plastic emesis basins that intrigue children because of their curvilinear shape are rarely at hand for sudden vomiting. So: count on helping to clean up if you are at the bedside for several days.

Unless someone's in an isolation unit, vomit is rarely infectious. For cosmetic or personal preferences, you may wish to wear gloves while cleaning up. {→Hands and Gloves.}

What you must watch for is the aftermath, in which some vomit may be swallowed back into the wrong airway and result in coughing or sensations of choking, which are not only frightening but can lead to →aspiration and stressful breathing.

We do not encourage vomiting as we did in the past, when the purpose of medicine was to get bad stuff out of the body by hook or by crook--using cathartics or purgatives, enemas, diuretics, hot sweats, blisters, expectorants, vomitories, cupping or leeching. Today, aside from the use of stomach pumps, we try to kill the bad stuff on-site and look to the body to expel the corpuscular corpses silently. So vomiting is more dramatic than ever, because less welcome.

Or not: the judges of beer-drinking and pie-eating contests take it as proof of serious effort; bulimics practice it ritually; pregnant women cope with it through traditional recipes. But it's surprisingly easy to wax philosophical about vomit. One blogger (a suspense novelist) has seen the meaning(lessness) of life in the manufacture of rubber blobs of fake vomit. From this it is the shortest of steps to Jean-Paul Sartre's existential novel, *Nausea*.

Where vomiting is frequent, there are anti-nausea preparations (the best, and most expensive, may be Zofran) but you can also try salted soda crackers, which absorb the liquid in the gut that contributes to the upsurge of vomit. If you become nauseous in the presence of another's nausea, salted crackers may help you too. One could build a new philosophy upon this sharing.

WAITING

Hours, days, weeks, months of waiting. At the bedside, you are always waiting for something: a doctor to call back; a pharmacy delivery to arrive; morphine to take effect; a home health aide to knock; a physical therapist to show up; morphine to take effect; lab results to be reported; laxatives to kick in; morphine to take effect; →respite.

There are good excuses for the delay, even at home, for each caregiver has limits on how much she can do, how quickly he can do it. So do floor nurses and the staff in medical offices, t pharmacists in drugstores, and lab technicians working through rush orders, all amid routine screw-ups in communication due to hastily scribbled telephone notes, or the confusion of changed orders, revised dosages, new treatment protocols.

And pain and morphine (or hydrocodone, or fentanyl) are ever in a battle of wills.

So there will be waiting. With waiting comes fantasy. Like people who while away their time in long lines by imagining themselves in exotic places, everyone in bed or at the bedside will have periods when their minds lift away from the run-of-the-mill toward the unreal or implausible. For the seriously ill and the Departing, these may become strong hallucinations. For you, vivid fictions. Write these down. Talk about them.

Waiting can be another form of →sitting. Over time, it can be a hazard, as you become such a doyen of waiting that you may be slow to recognize →emergencies, slow to respond to one more apparent crisis from which, doubtless, the "patient" (what a word!) will recover, with no medical intervention. Moreover, by now you will have hussled out to ERs so frequently that you are reluctant to subject anyone to another hurry-up-and-wait routine after the initial →triage. You know that few get out of an ER in under four hours; waiting for a hospital bed to open up can take hours more. And maybe your lethargic response is really spite, since you yourself are sick-and-tired of someone else being sick and tired (someone, for example, who is old and retired and has led a full life), and why wait another week or month or year for the final act?

It's not spite, but you have a ways to go in mastering the art of waiting. Take some deep breaths. Call a friend.

Alert!! Some hospitals will admit a patient from ER "for observation." Medicare and private insurance both balk at paying for such non-interventional hospital stays, so patients can end up being responsible for the entire hospital bill.

WALKERS

Beside almost every sickbed is a walker, folded up in a corner or standing in an empty aluminum embrace. Walkers have become an icon of the progression of illness from debility to departure, but the icon is misleading, for many of the seriously ill insist upon walking on their own until they are too frail to walk at all. However much they may →fear death, they seem to fear the walker more.

Some manage with walkers for years, like old tennis players still kicking at balls when they can no longer swing at them (or that's what it looks like, with those split tennis balls on the legs to cushion the tips).

But for those who used to jog miles each morning, the walker is a dread, dreary totem of loss. Loss not only of mobility but of motility, that is, of liveliness: a four-square replacement for a life that not long ago could pivot on an instant in most any arc. Walkers do not easily pivot and swing; a person must lift them up to make radical changes in direction. Walkers keep a person stable by limiting the capacity for swift shifts of momentum or focus. They are best at straight lines and level surfaces.

So the walker is in the corner not from benign neglect but from exile. Enough with plodding tours of a rectilinear world, say the seriously ill and Departing. Death is not made with T-squares. .

J. J. Hadamard, a French mathematician who worked on prime numbers and two-dimensional manifolds, asserted that "the shortest and best way between two truths of the real domain often passes through the imaginary one." Studying the nature and process of scientific insight, he found that many problems were solved by physicists and mathematicians who did not, as it were, use walkers to take one slow step after another until they reached a solution, but who saw the problem and solution as a spontaneous whole. They let their minds operate in the realm of the imaginary, through whose curves they cut a path from the well-known beyond the apparently insoluble.

You do not sit at the bedside to hold a person to the four-square. Those abed have primes, manifolds, and matrices of astonishing complexity and intrigue in their own history. How a person passes from life into death may be no less than a passage through the imaginary toward some solution you can only wonder at.

You sit at the bedside, then, not to help them up into a walker but to help them, as best you can, toward some spontaneous whole, an illumination at least of competence and wholeness as a human being, of what it takes to be *here*.

WEEPING

Weeping is semiotically unsteady. It means too many things, wells up from too many sources, spills over from too many constellations of emotions to be reliably comprehensible. At the bedside you are likely to weep, but no one can say why, or what the weeping will mean.

The Departing may weep on first receiving a terminal diagnosis, or on news of a last-ditch therapy denied or failed. They may weep throughout the months leading up to the Last Days. Weeping can also be a physiological →sign of the approaching end, tears issuing from the eyes as yet another penultimate form of release.

If you yourself have not wept during the Last Days, you may weep in the Days After, and not just during the funeral or memorial. Tears come on the →anniversaries of departures, years later.

Or, you may not weep. Not weeping is also semiotically unsteady, although there must be some gender conditioning at work where men rarely weep and women weep much {→Women and Men.}. Not weeping has little to do with a capacity for →grief. Trying to force tears because they are expected is peculiarly human, and peculiarly uncomfortable.

If you weep, accept the weeping. Do not stifle or suppress it.

If you do not weep, do not think any less of yourself.

Sobbing is something else. For many families (and sometimes for hospital or SNF staff), the heaving sounds of sobbing are unnerving, threatening. Sobbing is subject to being interpreted as the expression of shock, anger, or bitterness out of which may come bad relations, bad publicity, or costly litigation {→Lawyers}. Weeping is quieter than sobbing.

Children can be frightened by the weeping of adults, more frightened by sobbing. They need to be assured that they are not the cause of people bent over in tears or running out of a room. Confused and surprised by the drama around them, they themselves may start crying without knowing quite why, and for that reason their crying may go on inexplicably long, as if having a tantrum. Such crying is no tantrum. It must be acknowledged as genuine and under no circumstances explained away {→Young People}.

Each culture has its own approach to weeping, sobbing, wailing.

All human beings cry.

WILLS

Living Wills are not the same as Last Wills and Testaments, in that Living Wills do not specify the inheritors of the estate of the Departing, or who will get what. In making out a Living Will, or the popular Five Wishes booklet available from →Aging with Dignity, it may occur to the seriously ill or the Departing to make changes to an existing will, or to write a new one. A will composed informally can be acceptable in courts of law so long as it is signed in the presence of two witnesses who themselves are not designated inheritors of any part of the estate. The two witnesses sign as witnesses to the signature of the testator (will-maker); they need not read a word of the document, but they must date their signatures and print their names beneath, with their addresses.

For complex estates, complex last wishes, or feuding, litigious families, it is better to get the help of an attorney in drafting a will. (I am not an attorney. Nothing anywhere in this guide has legal standing.)

Preparing a will, on your own or with the help of an attorney, may speed up the legal settlement of an estate, especially if the estate is uncontested, but the estate must still go through probate unless valued under an amount differently determined by each state ($150,000, for example, in California). Since probate can take months in the simplest of circumstances, years if complicated, people often create family trusts, which sidestep probate. Material and advice about trusts can be found on the web, in any public library, at legal aid societies, and often at senior centers.

When notified of a death, the county coroner must decide whether an autopsy is necessary. An autopsy, with ensuing lab work, can delay probate proceedings for weeks or months. When the Departing is in →hospice, palliative care, or a →skilled nursing facility, it is unlikely that an autopsy will be required. To avoid autopsies, some choose ahead of time to donate their bodies at death to a hospital or medical school that will use them for clinical research or education in anatomy. Such programs will pick up the body at death, at no charge; some will return the (cremated) body when the research or educational program is complete (in a year or more), and some will not. Before signing on to an →organ donor program, religious and sentimental (cemetery) issues must be resolved, even where it is only a partial donor program (e.g., for →eyes or kidneys).

A while ago, the Departing used wills to reiterate their faith, state their expectations of survivors, impart wisdom to young fools, even to square accounts with a prodigal child This is rare now that we have such an armory of Living Wills, Organ Donor forms, Family Trusts, and other legal instruments for ensuring the performance of one's last wishes. But a new informal instrument is gaining appeal: →Ethical Wills.

To make or remake a will during the Last Days would not seem like a good idea, especially if the Departing's judgment is clouded by opiates or pain, but the desire to make a will can be understood as a final assertion of personal will or the last expression of a will to power over (anticipatory) others. Or the will to live on.

Willpower.
Will to power.
Will he won't he?
Willy-nilly.
Will o' the wisp.

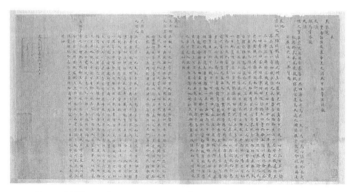

Last Will and Testament of the Kangxi Emperor
(1654-1722), fourth emperor of the Qing dynasty

WINDOWS

Pressed to name the most valuable benefit of being at home while seriously ill or Departing, I would say: windows. Windows that open. Windows whose blinds or curtains are under one's control. Windows with northern and southern exposures, with views out to the sunrise or sunset. Windows with trees beyond, birdfeeders and birds, flower gardens or forest, hills or mountains or, yes, cityscapes and fire escapes. Clear panes or stained glass, clerestories or French doors. Windows.

It's not just the →light. It's the kinaesthetics. With windows come sensations of movement: from the bed and bedside, throughout the day, a person can direct and redirect light and shadow, can feel the passage of sun and clouds, of wind through leaves and screens. Beyond, voices and forms pass close by or at a finite distance, but unlike the voices and forms in hospital or →SNF, these are unimpressed by illness, unconstrained by monitors, alarms, and rounds of meals and medicine. The openly windowed world is a world in play.

Oh, there are more windows than there used to be in hospitals and nursing homes, but they are rarely as amenable as those at home, and rarely can one plant as one wishes in the space beyond, or hang hummingbird feeders, or open them at exactly the best angle for the time of day, and change the angle from hour to hour.

The stars at →night, how often are they visible to patients in hospital? The moon?

And I would sing doubly the praises of windows for those at the bedside, who are often as much shut-in as those abed. At first it may be a pain to have to open and close windows, raise and lower blinds, spread and close curtains throughout the day, but soon you will find it a welcome form of physical and spiritual exercise, a reminder of wider environments that become endless topics of conversation: weather, climate, architecture, city planning, the history of rural and urban, where you both have come from, where you both have never been, where you would like to go, where you are most content, most inspired, most at peace.

Windows. At once too obvious and too expansive a metaphor of transparent presence, let them be whatever they become, each day, between both of you and the motions of the world beyond. Frames. Membranes. Pinholes. Spyglasses. Filters.

They are at your mercy.

WINNOWING (not the same as →Triage)

Weeks, months, years before the Long Days, the winnowing begins: years, when a widow/er moves to smaller quarters; months, when a family faces the likelihood of a departure; weeks, when space must be made for a hospital bed and other medical appliances {→Doodads} at home under hospice care.

Although it will seem rude to be sorting through possessions before departure, winnowing can often deepen the Last Months. As you go through desks, closets, garages, you will need to engage those abed in order to make sense of what it is you've found. You'll learn things about the seriously ill you had never thought to ask or the Departing to share. For those who have little, it's doubly important to ask about what they've managed to hold close {→Keepsakes}. Why did my friend Sandra, a Jewish bohemian throughout her life, have at the end only a small Isfahan prayer rug and her marriage certificate?

You are not likely to finish the winnowing before departure, but in the Days After it will be emotionally harder to continue, as the simplest scrap of paper or odd button feels like a memento.

Some guidelines for winnowing, at any stage:

For safekeeping in a fireproof box: immigration/naturalization papers; birth certificates; military discharge papers; stock certificates and bonds; life insurance policies; social security card; trust or will; last 3 years of tax filings; recent bank statements; patents; warranties still in effect. You'll need access to these in the Days After, so remember where you put them. (Death certificates should also go in here.)
For shredding: bank, stock, and social security statements and receipts more than a year old-- or 3 years if significant; credit cards; Medicare card. It's your call on the passport.
To save for survivors or archives: photos; journals; original art/music/poetry/scholarship; voice/video recordings; military memorabilia; letters and cards of moment (no Get Well cards unless signed by the famous or famously reclusive); family bibles; diplomas; family trees; prestigious awards; diplomas.
To give to charity or thrift stores: whatever no one else wants that's still in good (working) condition--clothing, jewelry, clocks, watches, furniture, linens, cookware, dishes, books, CDs, music players, semi-antiques {→Recycling}.

What are the most problematic? Amateur sports trophies; non-military ribbons or medals; certificates of appreciation. Unless you intend to build a shrine, these have no place, yet you know how dear these were to the Departing. Or you have no clue.

WIVES, HUSBANDS, AND LOVERS

Long departures entail the past. The longer the departure, the more probably an ex will appear. With high divorce rates, blended families, and the complexities of modern cohabiting, departures can entangle those at the bedside in a maze of relationships ancient and current.

This can happen when the Departing is in her nineties and at last revealing that she is a lesbian, or eighty and insisting that the young woman of sixty-seven he has recently been seeing be granted primary status at the bedside, in preference to kin.

It is as much depth as length of relationship that counts toward the assigning of roles at the bedside. A wife, husband, or lover may feel called upon to reaffirm the depth of her love, the extent of his devotion. Others may invoke archaic good times in the face of a receding present and narrowed future. There will be unavoidable regret for trips cancelled, medical avenues blocked or unexplored, conversations interrupted.

Faithfulness is such a prominent issue at the end that it can be mistaken for love. Conversely, if a (healthy) spouse is not attending devotedly to the Departing, this may be mistaken for indifference, or a love grown stale, when instead it may be →grief, or fear of being alone in the Days After, or →fatigue.

Where a husband, wife, or lover is the principal →caregiver, there will be times of frustration or anger at having to spend one's days like this. Old habits of mutual miscommunication, nagging, or competitiveness ("you think *you're* suffering?") do not disappear simply because the Last Months are turning toward the Last Days. {Consider →Mutual Peril.}

Long-time lovers, especially those not named in Advance →Directives or →Powers of Attorney, may find themselves having to prove themselves yet again to family, as well as to hospital staff and visiting nurses. They may stake their claim to a place at the bedside by assuming the most grueling or distasteful of tasks. Meanwhile they may find themselves stifling their own grief or hostility in order to appear particularly loving and worthy of the respect of family and friends

Husbands and wives may resent all those fluttering around the bedside {→Gatekeeping.}. Or they may resent the demands of the Departing, after years of having labored as a couple toward a mutual independence. Of course, they will tell no one about these feelings. That would be unseemly.

How very much of the Last Days gets caught up, to no avail, in concerns about the unseemly.

WOMEN AND MEN

Because they live on average several years longer than men. . . because they have traditionally taken on, or been trapped in, the role of →caregiving. . . because they have customarily been trained as →nurses rather than physicians or chemists, despite millennia of skill as healers and herbalists. . . because they have been thought to possess a tender touch, soothing voice, infinite patience. . . and because, until recently, they have been the chief cooks, maids, and bottle-washers: women have had more experience at bedsides than men.

The majority of nurses, hospice nurses and volunteers are women, as are home health aides. At the bedside daily the only men you are likely to encounter are orderlies and physical or respiratory therapists. Men take care of the past tense: undertakers, funeral directors. It is poorly-paid women who deal with the day-to-day →pain, →vomit, and →anxiety, and who know how to change the bedsheets of the frail and the frightened.

Because of all this, do women conduct their own departures differently than men? Do they deal with pain differently? Do they want more company? Less? Do they need different drugs or a different rhetoric for the Last Days? Surely the departure of a woman takes on a different trajectory than that of a man, so must be differently accompanied, attended to, understood?

Few such distinctions appear in the literature on end-of-life care. Apparently, dying is not as gendered as is Death, who in the West is female when seducing toward dissolution or suicide (the *femme fatale*), male when collecting bodies (the mortician in his dark suit with his black hearse) and souls (that hooded figure with the deep voice and dark robes). Somehow, during the Last Days our years of having learned to lead a life as a man or woman seem to drop away toward the neuter, ashes to ashes, passions to passionless.

There is something appealing about such gender neutrality, as if on the advance of age and the approach of death each body returns to undifferentiated cells. There is also something very disturbing, for to ignore a lifetime of gendered experience is to ignore much of who the Departing has become over the years. Recording a woman's history during the Last Months, how strange it would sound were the Departing never to make mention of a gendered role (→mother or daughter, aunt or niece), never express a gendered sexual desire. Is gender such a ghostly raiment that it is best unhooked from our bones on the way out?

X'S

Unknowns stand at every crossroads of the Last Months and Last Days:

What was the original cause (the remote etiology) of this terminal illness?
Unknown.

How did an acute condition became chronic, then fatal?
Can't rightly say...{→Cascades; Depression; Iatrogenesis; Signs}.

Why can he remember this but not that?
How can she be failing yet so clear-headed?
Neurologists themselves have no idea...{→Consciousness; Forgetfulness}.

When will the Departing depart?
Oh, soon...{→Buying Time; ETD; Readiness; Signs}

How can doctors who are so unwilling or unable to tell you about near futures be so confident of their profession and so sure of themselves?
Guess...{→Physicians and Surgeons}

How are you going to feel after the departure?
How will your sister cope?
Will your father be able to live by himself?
Time will tell...{→Anniversaries; Grieving; Mortal Peril}.

Who are these people showing up unannounced, all these unfamiliar faces?
Ex's: ex-wives, ex-husbands, ex-mothers-in-law, ex-boy friends, former cellmates, first loves from high school, fiancé(e)s abandoned at the altar, people you have never met, never heard of, or never wanted to see again....Ex/tension.

Bones glow under x-rays but the sixty per cent of us that is water is invisible to x-rays, a metaphor for all that remains unrevealed in the Last Days.

Radiophotographically and philosophically, Death may be an ending without full resolution. The Departing does not have all the answers, and in extremis does not need all the answers. Nor will you.

YELLOW PADS

Tired from hours at the bedside, trying to maintain a semblance of your own life, you may not feel much like writing, but there are good reasons to keep pens and a pad of paper with you. Why?

•To record memos, questions, or recollections.
•To take down →physicians' and surgeons' explanations, their proposed courses of treatment, names of new→medications.
•To note phone messages and visitors who have come at the wrong time.
•To leave messages for visitors, →caregivers, or →nurses while you are off at lunch (and please, go to lunch. Take a walk.)
•To keep track of medical mistakes, hospital or SNF screw-ups {→Advocacy, Iatrogenesis}..
•To formulate →questions about care, prospective care, or legal or ethical issues that have arisen in the course of the day.
•To make lists of errands, people to call, things to get.
•To keep track of the contact numbers of →hospice or hospital staff, pharmacies, therapists, →social workers, visiting nurses, →case managers, referrals, and so forth.

And to write up what you are thinking, feeling, and fearing to think or feel or say, each day. Some people keep diaries all of their lives. Some go through a spurt of journaling when they are looking for answers at difficult junctures in their lives. Some write long e-mails or frequent text messages instead, because they think of writing as signaling. In whatever manner, and for whatever number of minutes you can manage, it's useful to write about what you are thinking, feeling, hoping.

Writing is never merely a repetition of what you are thinking; as you write, the words report back to you, and you reflect on them in order to move on, or you find yourself able to move on precisely because the words are reporting back. Without writing, you lose out on a means of communion that is at once private and revealing. The words may look ungainly, all scratched out, circled, or rearranged with arrows and dotted lines, but they are your words, and you need them.

For all of these purposes, yellow pads are particularly useful because they are easily indexed along the margins and harder to misplace than slips of paper, pages torn from magazines, or the backs of flyers. Be sure to put your name and phone number on the top taped edge, in case you do misplace a pad. (Ditto, or approximately ditto, for an I-pad , laptop, or tablet.)

YOU'LL BE THE DEATH OF ME

Deadbolts, deadlocks, dead-ends . . . the English language is blithe with death. We no longer use dying as a synonym for orgasm, as in the time of Shakespeare and Ben Jonson, but a person can still be "dead right," "dead-set against," even "dead to the world," yet nowhere near the Last Days.

Likely you'll let slip with one of these phrases while at the bedside. You'll scarcely be aware of it until a friend suggests that maybe you shouldn't talk about a certain chef's salad being something "to die for."

Deadbeats, deadwood, dead letters, deadpan faces . . . so much death, dead-center in our daily discourse.

So what? Am I supposed to change the way I speak just because I'm at the bedside?

In fact, you do change the way you speak when you're at the bedside, at least at the beginning, and when a situation seems desperate {→Acuteness, Urgency}. You tend not to speak as loudly or as quickly, and to pause more often. You tend to use shorter sentences. You tend to ask questions that come out of nowhere, because at the bedside you do not say everything you are thinking, so the logical connections go unspoken.

Death's-head spiders, the Dead Sea, the Grateful Dead. . . .

Are you telling me that I should be censoring the allusions I make and idioms I use? Should my death-words come solely in the context of dead-serious conversations about entering →hospice, ending a lifelong feud, debating the →risk of a surgery, contacting a prodigal daughter?

No, you don't have to be so cautious. The cautiousness itself would be more upsetting than any deathly slips of the tongue.

There is, however, one phrase you might think twice about. "Dead weight." As the end nears, the Departing do become dead weight. They cannot lift themselves up, cannot help with the lifting or turning of their bodies. They may be paralyzed, they may be weak, they may be drugged, they may be unwilling (because of the pain), or they may simply want to be left alone. Dead weight is heavy with consequence.

Then there's "death-defying," a P.-T.-Barnum sort of phrase, a wonderland idiom, and although each moment of life in an entropic universe is literally death-defying, it does not seem apt either as encouragement or expectation during the Last Days. Why not? You tell me. I could be dead wrong.

YOUNG PEOPLE

Young people will want to know details you think are too stark or gruesome, which is why parents and theologians have recourse to afterstories of the passage of souls, reincarnations or celestial rejoinings. But the young will still want to know what happens to the body, which is what they have been trying to figure out since they were born--what happens if I do this, or that, to my physical world. And they are not squeamish.

They are also often fine at the bedside, though inconstant. They cannot →sit for long. They can hold hands and be quiet, or tell a wandering story. They can listen for a while, even to gibberish. And they like being appreciated as one of the group who have come to the bedside.

Engaged, they will be →sad but not forever, and not at a loss for what to say. They will run errands, take out the dog, have serious conversations or, when older, short exchanges of black humor {→Jokes, Laughter}.

Excluded from the bedside, they will blame you forever and then some. They will wonder what they did to deserve to be shut out, or why the Departing did not want to see them. They know about death, in some sense, and if younger children ask when a parent or grandparent or aunt is coming back home months afterwards, they ask in part because the physics of death is still mystifying: they have not accepted it as a spiritual mystery or a material finality. Neither have many adults.

It is doubly important for them to be invited to the bedside when a friend or close cousin their own age is about to die. There will be tears, anger, and some recurrent →anxiety (Am I next? Was I responsible?). But keeping them away will only compound the tears, anger, and anxiety.

Very young children require honesty also, but they do not need all of the medical details. They will know, however, when you or the doctors are perplexed or in suspense.

Children and teenagers must →grieve differently than adults, for they have different anchors in time. They may play out their grief in music or art, in dance or story. The young must know from us that they too have something to contribute to the Last Days, something that would be missing if they were not there. We need them from start to finish, always.

ZERO VISIBILITY

Deep in, the Long Days threaten to become a cave where you can see only an inch or two in front of you. Focus narrows and strains; your steps become smaller, more tentative; you don't know when a wall will give way or the roof angle down.

This is not a description of the experiences of the Departing. It is a description of the experiences of those at the bedside who become so lost in the process of a friend's illness or beloved's departure that there are no other horizons. You may use other metaphors: winter fog, arctic night, sandstorm, black hole.

For people at the bedside who have their own health problems or have been battling →depression, zero visibility may come on fast and dangerously. For others, even the most resilient, fog or sandstorm is ever looming, all the more so when it is a child or a young adult who is departing.

Nearness-unto-death can become, under conditions of zero visibility, a state of near-death. You do not want that. Empathy with the Departing does not entail wearing a death mask. Indeed, the seriously ill and the Departing want, as long as possible, to be looking outward. There is only so much sick-talk one can take before one wants to feel the sun, make a →joke, be of help.

Yes, the Departing often choose gestures or tones of voice or sparse words that they believe will be helpful to those around them. Or they keep silent if silence will help. So long as they are aware and under no insurmountable pain, the Departing want to be engaged as more than subjects of a preliminary mourning. Some want to plan their funerals or wakes, some want to give technical advice on buying a house or a computer, some want to make art; most of them also want to help others. There is frequently a rare kindness to the Last Days, as self-importance diminishes and grudges dissipate {→Grumps}.

Do not dismiss the inclination of the Departing to want to be of help. Do not say, No, this is your time, tell us what you want and we'll make it happen, don't worry about us. It is human to worry about others, to want to help them; it can be how we define ourselves as essentially human.

Zero visibility around those at the bedside tends to close down this avenue for the expression of the best part of ourselves even as it makes it harder for the Departing to lend a word, a hand, a smile, a wink, or the warmth of a finger's touch.

Focus for clarity, for presence, but keep your hands in the world. With theirs.

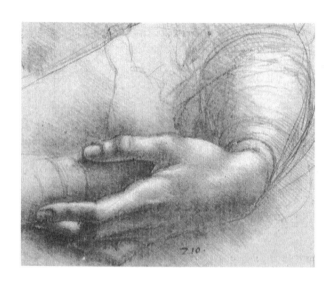

FURTHER READING

Beauvoir, Simone de. *A Very Easy Death*, trans. Patrick O'Brian (Pantheon, 1985).

Bell, Karen Whitley. *Living at the End of Life: A Hospice Nurse Addresses the Most Common Questions* (Sterling, 2010).

Bonanno, George A. *The Other Side of Sadness: What the New Science of Bereavement Tells Us about Life after Loss* (Basic, 2009).

Brody, Jane, *Guide to the Great Beyond: Prepare Now for a Smooth Ride to the End of Life* (Random House, 2009).

Bruera, Eduardo et al. *Textbook of Palliative Medicine* (Hodder Arnold, 2006).

Byock, Ira. *The Best Care Possible: A Physician's Quest to Transform Care Through the End of Life*. (Avery, 2012). and many others

Callanan, Maggie. *Final Journeys: A Practical Guide for Bringing Care and Comfort at the End of Life* (Bantam, 2008).

Callanan, Maggie and Patricia Kelley. *Final Gifts: Understanding the Special Awareness, Needs, and Communications of the Dying* (Bantam, 1997).

Cappello, Mary. *Called Back: My Reply to Cancer, My Return to Life* (Alyson, 2009).

Coberly, Margaret. *Sacred Passage: How to Provide Fearless, Compassionate Care for the Dying* (Shambhala, 2003).

Colby, William. *The Long Goodbye* (Hay House, 2003).

Didion, Joan. *The Year of Magical Thinking* (Knopf, 2005; audio, Highbridge, 2006).

Dolan, Susan, and Audrey Vizzard, *The End of Life Advisor: Personal, Legal, and Medical Considerations for a Peaceful, Dignified Death* (Kaplan, 2008).

Dresser, Norine, and Freda Wasserman. *Saying Goodbye to Someone You Love* (Demos Medical, 2010).

Faull, Christina et al., eds. *Handbook of Palliative Care*, 2nd ed. (Blackwell, 2005).

Feldman, David B. and Stephen A. Lasher, Jr., *The End of Life Handbook: A Compassionate Guide to Connecting with and Caring for a Dying Loved One* (New Harbinger, 2008).

Gerberg, Mort, ed. *Last Laughs: Cartoons about Aging, Retirement . . . and the Great Beyond* (Scribners, 2007).

Glaser, Barney G. and Anselm L. Strauss. *Time for Dying* (Aldine, 1968).

Glenn, Evelyn N. *Forced to Care: Coercion and Caregiving in America* (Harvard, 2010).

Gutkind, Lee, ed. *At the End of Life: True Stories about How We Die* (In Fact, 2012).

FURTHER READING, continued

Gutkind, Lee, ed. *Twelve Breaths a Minute: End of Life Essays* (SMU, 2011).

Hammes, Bernard. *Having Your Own Say: Getting the Right Care When It Matters Most* (Gundersen Lutheran, 2012).

Hart, Julian Tudor. "Inverse Care Law," *Lancet* 1 (1971) pp. 405-12.

Humphrey, Derek. *Final Exit: The Practicalities of Self Deliverance and Assisted Suicide for the Dying* (Hemlock Society, 1991).

Hutchinson, Joyce, and Joyce Rupp. *May I Walk You Home? Courage and Comfort for Caregivers of the Very Ill* (Ave Maria, 1999/2009).

Justin, Renate, "At the end of life, do we need to hide?" *Annals of Long-Term Care* 13 (Nov 2005), available online at: www.annalsoflongtermcare.com/article/4932

Kessler, David. *The Needs of the Dying: A Guide for Bringing Hope, Comfort, and Love to Life's Final Chapter* (Harper, 2007).

Kessler, David. *Visions, Trips, and Crowded Rooms: What You See Before You Die* (Hay House, 2011).

Karnes, Barbara. *Gone from My Sight: The Dying Experience* (Barbara Karnes Books, POB 822139, Vancouver WA 98682).

Kiernan, Stephen P. *Last Rights: Rescuing the End of Life from the Medical System* (St. Martin's, 2007).

Kinzbrunner, Barry M. et al. *20 Common Problems in End-of-Life Care* (McGraw-Hill, 2002).

Kittay, Eva F. *Love's Labor: Essays on Women, Equality, and Dependency* (Routledge, 1999).

Kübler-Ross, Elisabeth. *On Death and Dying* (Macmillan, 1969).

Kuhl, David. *What Dying People Want* (Public Affairs, 2003).

Lynn, Joanne, and Joan Harrold. *A Handbook for Mortals. Guidance for People Facing Serious Illness* (Oxford, 1999)

Miller, James E. and Susan Cutshall. *The Art of Being a Healing Presence* (Willowgreen, 2001).

Paolini, Charlotte A. "Symptoms Management at the End of Life," *Journal of the American Osteopathic Association* 101 (Oct 2001), pp. 609-15, online at www.jaoa.org/cgi/reprint/101/10/609.pdf

Pipher, Mary. *Another Country: Navigating the Emotional Terrain of Our Elders* (Riverhead, 1999).

Randall, Fiona and R. S. Downie. *The Philosophy of Palliative Care* (Oxford, 2006).

Schneiderman, Lawrence J. *Embracing Our Mortality: Hard Choices in an Age of Medical Miracles* (Oxford, 2008).

FURTHER READING, continued

Smith, Douglas C. *Caregiving: Hospice Proven Techniques for Healing Body and Soul* (Wiley, 1997)

Span, Paula. *When the Time Comes: Families With Aging Parents Share Their Struggles and Solutions* (Grand Central Life & Style, 2009)

Spark, Muriel. *Memento Mori* (Penguin, 1959, later editions).

Terman, Stanley A., with Ronald B. Miller and Michael S. Evans. *The Best Way to Say Goodbye: A Legal Peaceful Choice at the End of Life* (Life Transitions, 2007).

Trillin, Calvin. *About Alice* (Random House, 2006, also e-book).

Verghese, Abraham, "The Smell of Death," in *My Own Country: A Doctor's Story* (Vintage, 1994); also as "The Odor of Death" at www.ralphmag.org/verghese.html

Webb, Marilyn. *The Good Death: The New American Search to Reshape the End of Life* (Bantam, 1999), on the right-to-die movement.

"What is a good death?" *British Medical Journal* (BMJ) 327 (2003) pp. 173-237.

White, Patrick, *Eye of the Storm* (Viking, 1974).

Wicks, Robert J. *Overcoming Secondary Stress in Medical and Nursing Practice: A Guide to Professional Resilience and Personal Well Being* (Oxford, 2005).

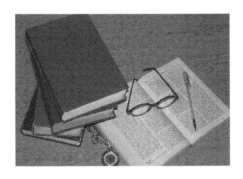

Further Viewing/Listening: FILMS, PLAYS, RADIO, VIDEO

Bensted, Anna, and Rachel Botbaum, reporters. "Quality of Death, End of Life Care in America" (Inside Out, WBUR, 2009). Listen at http://insideout.wbur.org/documentaries/qualityofdeath/#

Benton, Donna. "Respite Care: Caring for the Caregiver" (Wiland Bell /Aquarius, 2004). Dr. Benton of USC's Andrus School of Gerontology, on safeguarding caregivers.

Cantor, Karen and Chris Gavin. *Last Rights: Facing End-of-Life Choices* (Singing Wolf Documentaries, 2009).

Duke, Trish. *Dying to Live* (2012). Four episodes bring us "into the homes of patients and families who openly share how they faced the rollercoaster ride from diagnosis through the progression of a terminal disease."

Edson, Margaret. *Wit* (Dramatists Play Service, 1999). The final hours of a woman who has been a literature professor and is now dying of ovarian cancer.

Four Corners, ABC Australia, producer Janine Cohen. *Final Call* (Journeyman Pictures, 2007). On the death-with-dignity movement, at www.journeyman.tv/?lid'57477&tmpl'transcript

Front Line, producers Miri Navasky and Karen O'Connor. "Facing Death" (PBS, 2010-11). Five segments at www.pbs.org/wgbh/pages/frontline/facing-death/

Henderson, Lily F., and Shana Hashaviah. *Lessons for the Living* (Fantasia, 2010). Documentary on hospice patients and caregivers.

Hill, Mike (dir.) and Sue Collins (prod.). *Life Before Death* (Moonshine Films, 2011). Follows health care professionals in 11 countries battling "the sweeping epidemic of pain that threatens to condemn one in every ten of us to an agonizing and shameful death." Raises awareness about hospice and palliative care. Supported by the Lien Foundation. See www.lifebeforedeath.com/movie/watch the movie.shtml

Kaldhusdal, Terry and Michael Bernhagen. *Consider the Conversation: A Documentary on a Taboo Subject* (Burning Hay Wagon Productions, 2011). On euthanasia, right to die.

KBTC Documentaries, "In My Time of Dying" (2011). Interviews with medical experts and spiritual leaders, interwoven with portraits of people facing death.

Moyers, Bill. *On Our Own Terms* (WNET New York, PBS, 2000), and see www.pbs.org/wnet/onourownterms/tools/index.html

Russell, Charlie and Terry Pratchett, producer/director. *Choosing to Die* (KEO North for BBC Scotland/ BBC Two, 2011). Interview at http://vimeo.com/25239708.

For more documentary films: www.aquariusproductions.com

USEFUL (not-for-profit) WEBSITES

AARP (American Association of Retired People):
www.aarp.org/families/end_life A rich resource with
information also on wills and power of attorney

Aging with Dignity: www.agingwithdignity.org,
for Five Wishes living will ($5)

American Association for Clinical Chemistry:
www.labtestsonline.org
on understanding lab tests and results, with baselines.

American Hospice Foundation: www.americanhospice.org

American Psychological Association:
www.apa.org/pi/aids/programs/eol/index.aspx

Canadian Hospice Palliative Care Organization: www.chpca.net

Caregiver Resource Network, www.caregiverresource.net

Center for Applied Ethics and Professional Practice,
www2.edc.org/lastacts, an archive of 28 thematic issues on
Innovations in End-of-Life Care (1999-2003)

Center for Gerontology, Brown University Medical School,
"Toolkit of Instruments to Measure End-of-Life Care,"
www.chcr.brown.edu/pcoc/Physical.htm

Chicago End-of-Life Care Coalition, www.cecc.info/resource

Family Caregiver Alliance,
www.caregiver.org/caregiver/jsp/home.jsp

Green Burials, www.greenburials.org, for biodegradable caskets

Greenhouse Project, http://thegreenhouseproject.org, which
aims to return people to the community in small homes
offering a full range of care and clinical services.

Growthhouse & Inter-Institutional Collaborating Network
On End Of Life Care, www.growthhouse.org/iicn.html
for a free, shared database of 4000 pages on end-of-life care
from forty organizations in North America and Europe.

International Observatory on End of Life Resources, fine articles
and bibliography at
www.lancs.ac.uk/shm/research/ioelc/publications/

Lymphoma information, www.lymphomation.org.

Missouri End-of-Life Coalition, Guidelines for End-of-Life Care in
Long-Term Care Facilities (2003)
http://health.mo.gov/safety/showmelongtermcare

--also at Senior Health Knowledge Network,
www.shrtn.on.ca/node/1455

National Cancer Institute, National Institutes of Health,
www.cancer.gov/cancertopics/factsheet/Support/end-of-life-
care

USEFUL (not-for-profit) WEBSITES, continued

National Family Caregivers Association,
www.thefamilycaregiver.org, which "educates, supports, and
speaks up for the ... 65 million Americans who care for loved
ones with a chronic illness or disability or frailties of old age."

National Library of Medicine:
www.nlm.nih.gov/medlineplus/endoflifeissues.html

Pallipedia: http://pallipedia.org, an online dictionary of
palliative care terms.

POLST forms: www.ohsu.edu/polst/index.htm

Precious Legacy: a free-access e-book by Alan D. Lieberson,
Treatment of Pain and Suffering in the Terminally Ill (1999),
at www.preciouslegacy.com

Programs for the Elderly, at
www.programsforelderly.com/documentaries death.php

Pubmed, for up-to-date research on medical issues:
www.ncbi.nlm.nih.gov/pubmed

US government website for caregiver resources:
www.usa.gov/Citizen/Topics/Health/caregivers.shtml

Wong-Baker FACES Pain Rating Scale:
www.partnersagainstpain.com/printouts/A7012AS6.pdf

See also the websites of societies and associations working on
behalf of those with specific diseases or conditions, such as
adult-onset asthma, AIDS, ALS, Alzheimer's, breast cancer,
diabetes, fibromyalgia, heart disease, leukemia, lupus, multiple
myeloma, multiple sclerosis, paraplegia, Parkinson's, polio
survivors, prostate cancer, renal failure.

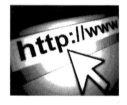

INDEX

Note: Since the text is arranged alphabetically by topic, and since each topic is addressed in a one- or two-page chapter, this index is meant rather to identify terms or phrases absent from--but implicit in--particular chapters. I also list relevant words or concepts one might not think to search for, and I provide references within the Index to synonyms or related ideas. Finally, I list drugs by both generic and trade names.

INDEX, Dignity-Expiration Dates

INDEX, Neurology-Physician Orders

INDEX, Unfairness-Writing

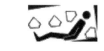

explained at: Bedsores

NOTE-TAKING & NOTE-MAKING*

*Or doodling. According to Jackie Andrade in "What Does Doodling Do?" *Applied Cognitive Psychology* (2009), doodling improves attention and recall.

53187955R00145

Made in the USA
San Bernardino, CA
08 September 2017